D0462334

PRIVATE
PRACTICE
HANDBOOK

"**I** do not like (nor have I ever written) testimonials, but, your book has helped incredibly!. . .I have never started a business or ever realized *all* that is involved in opening an office. Thank you for the help. I honestly think I would have pulled out my hair without it!"

—*Rick Jacobs, M.A., MFCC*
Private Practice,
Ashland, Oregon

"Although I have been in private practice more than 25 years, I found many of your ideas in PRIVATE PRACTICE HANDBOOK stimulating, valuable, and useful reminders."

—*Leonard Blank, Ph.D.*
Private Practice,
Princeton, New Jersey

"The timing of this book is a sign for me. . .It carries a message of understanding, encouragement and hope."

—*Dave Hartenberger, D.Min.*
Pastoral Counselor,
Portland, Oregon

"Two years ago I opened my private practice in Southern California. Before actually starting practice, I read your book, "Private Practice Handbook," from cover to cover. Your book is a *blueprint for success* in private practice and a constant source for referral information. . .I am pleased to report that my practice is running smoothly and successfully! Thank you for your book.

—*Donna S. Mognett, M.A., MFCC*
Private Practice,
Covina, California

"I have looked for years for a book like *Private Practice Handbook.* Finally, someone has taken the time to digest, analyze and organize all the myriad of details one must consider in private practice. During my professional career as an industrial psychologist I have dreamed of starting my own practice, but didn't know where to begin. This book takes it from "A" to "Z" and leaves nothing to chance. . .I have shared the *Handbook* with many colleagues and friends and it becomes more difficult to get back each time it's borrowed. It should be required reading in every graduate psychology program. . ."

—*Kenneth A. Pilone, M.A.*
Industrial Relations Manager,
TRW Corporation
Redondo Beach, California

"As a psychologist working in a hospital setting as well as having a private practice I found your book PRIVATE PRACTICE HANDBOOK to be a very easy-to-read practical guide to the development and maintenance of a private psychological practice. Your many ideas and sound wisdom has not only motivated me to pursue new avenues toward the expansion of my practice but has also given me the "how-to's" in simple language.

—*Frederick L. Gross, Ph.D.*
Director, Mental Health Unit,
Palmdale General Hospital,
Palmdale, California

"I made my decision to go into full-time private practice after 12 years of university teaching. I had debated the issue for several years but had no place within the university community to really learn about private practice. The information contained in PRIVATE PRACTICE HANDBOOK gave me not only concrete suggestions regarding office space, referral sources, fees, but also asked some provocative questions. . .I believe that anyone considering full-time private practice needs all the information, all the ideas and all the help he or she can get. I recommend that they include PRIVATE PRACTICE HANDBOOK in their resource material."

—*DeLoss D. Friesen, Ph.D.*
Private Practice
Beaverton, Oregon

"This is an eminently practical book with considerable experience behind it. It contains many sound suggestions, that someone inexperienced in private practice would hardly think of, especially in the area of how to set up a practice, how to get referrals, and how to maintain the practice. This book is a valuable asset for any therapist considering part time practice. The experienced professional will surely also find much that is useful in this book."

—*Louis Cooper, Ph.D.*
Veterans' Administration Hospital,
Tomah, Wisconsin

PRIVATE PRACTICE HANDBOOK

The Tools, Tactics & Techniques
For Successful Practice Development

SECOND EDITION

by

Charles H. Browning, Ph.D.

3662 Katella Avenue, Suite 218
Los Alamitos, California 90720

Private Practice Handbook

Second Edition Copyright © 1982 by Duncliff's International

All rights reserved, including the right to reproduce this book, or portions thereof, in any form, except for the inclusion of brief quotations in a review. All inquiries should be addressed to Duncliff's International, 3662 Katella Avenue, Suite 218, Los Alamitos, California 90720. This book was manufactured in The United States of America.

First Printing – January 1979
Second Printing – April 1982
Third Printing – February 1983

ISBN 0-911663-01-0

To—
A true partner, and best friend;
My inspiration, and co-heir to
the grace of life.
To my loving wife — B.J.

And To—
Adam

FOREWORD TO THE SECOND EDITION

While cleaning out his desk drawers in his office, a psychologist ran across an old shoe repair ticket. To the best of his recollection, he couldn't remember for the life of him anything about the shoes. It must have been several years ago that he had gotten this ticket.

Anyway, he stuck the ticket in his pocket, and after seeing nine patients, he headed home. On the way home he decided to stop off at the shoe repair shop. He walked up to the counter, handed the ticket to the old shoemaker, and, like a good psychologist, he didn't say a word.

The old gentleman studied the ticket for several moments, walked into the back room, came out, and with a confident nod to the good doctor, he said, "They'll be ready next Tuesday!"

It's been three long years since the First Edition was published and it seems that clinicians are becoming more and more inventive and business-wise these days. We've spent three years collecting their "blueprints of success" in the desk drawer. We finally got out the ticket and took it in for redemption. We assembled all the "brain-children" of our creative colleagues that they have proven to be winners, and quit procrastinating. You have in your hands the fruits of those labors.

You never know what's going to happen when you clean out your desk! Enjoy this fresh, new assortment of "the Best of the Best." You'll find the major changes in Chapters 11 and 12. But please remember . . .

The best book is the book that makes you want to put it down and think for yourself. The most successful ideas are those that have not yet been tried . . . YOURS!

C.H.B.
January, 1982

PREFACE

How To Manage A Successful Restaurant . . . How To Succeed in The Retail Grocery Business . . . How To Run A Thriving Gasoline Station . . . How To Raise Minks For Profit . . . How To Make A Million In Mail Order . . . ad infinitum . . .

We have "How To" books, manuals, handbooks, guides and workbooks on just about every kind of known business and professional activity under the sun. Those enterprising souls who have learned the "secrets" of the care and feeding of a successful professional or business venture have set down their wisdom in print for anyone who would care to apply it.

Can we say the same thing of those therapists who have "somehow" built booming private practices in their communities? Are the secrets of the successful practice detailed in black and white for the psychologist, who, tired of the classroom, the "publish or perish" treadmill, would like to break free of the system and set up his own practice? Or the graduate student, who, after spending years of his life buried in the stacks and under the trauma of the dissertation dilemma, would love to make his dreams come true in an office of his own — but doesn't know the first step in finding one? Or even the well-seasoned, vintage-old-timer who, long established in his own practice, wonders why it just lopes along, barely paying the bills, and void of excitement — where can he turn?

"Some fine day, when I've learned the ins-and-outs, nuts-and-bolts, the "secrets" that seem to be safely guarded — some day when they are no longer secrets to me I shall sit down and write a book. In that little book I'll list them one by one, recipe by recipe as one would if writing a cookbook, for those, my fellow colleagues, my friends, so that they might avoid my mistakes and apply those strategies that are tried and true. Some day I'll do all I can to shed some light on those secrets for the good of my colleagues and for the public at large."

That someday is today! This is that book!

There are some fine books in print today dealing with the very practical issues of running a private mental health practice. And we see seminars cropping up and workshops at conventions appearing more and more. And yet the emphasis seems to be still a bit too general. Issues such as insurance, scheduling, accounting methods, and time management are certainly important. But what one question does the eager therapist ask in his zeal to build his own practice? Nine times out of ten this is his query; "Just exactly how do I go about getting referrals, getting patients so that I can pay the insurance, have something to account, and have someone to schedule?" Another question asked by the more experienced clinician is this; "Are there specific ways that I can use my practice to generate additional income over and above that resulting from consultation with patients?"

The definite answers to these questions comprise the "secrets" that I have referred to; and make up the life-blood of this book.

At times while assembling this manual I have had an uneasy feeling. Because the "secrets" have been such sacred cows and privileged information for so long, I have experienced an eerie sense that somehow I was engaged in a kind of professional "industrial espionage." Suddenly in bold print appeared ideas and methods that were practiced every day. But till now they had been unspoken, understood and covert strategies that one "does not discuss openly." Or does he?

He does . . . and we shall!

In spite of my paranoia and perhaps some of the objections that will arise from the esoteric wing of our profession, I make no apology for unveiling the secrets for you. My only regret is that I have waited so long to get this material into your hands!

With that longwinded overture, let me now, if I may, address you to whom this handbook is directed.

To You, The Newcomer to Private Practice

I am especially excited for you as you approach your new enterprise. I remember the thrill of that first patient, that first office, the name on the door sign, and that first check. I also recall with less enthusiasm that long period of waiting for that first patient, the office that was so tough to find, and the bills that piled up on my desk! But that's why this handbook was written. So that you might bypass some of my struggles — and nightmares — to find smoother sailing toward success.

I know that you will be eager to jump in to those chapters on getting referrals and generating income from the practice. But a word of friendly advice, if you please:

Spend time (don't be in a hurry) in Chapters 1, 2, 3 and 10. This is the material out of which you'll build the foundation for your practice. And the practice is only as sure as its foundation! So take your time in these chapters, you'll be glad you did.

To You, My Fellow "Old-Timer"

If you're at all like me, you will likely dive headlong into Chapter 4, "How To Gain Recognition In Your Community." Time is at a premium, I know all too well. And you want to get your teeth into the "meat" of this book. That's fine and you can, if you wish, skip the first two chapters. You've been there before, I'm sure.

On the other hand, let me strongly urge you to do one thing before getting your hands on the nitty gritty.

It has doubtless been some time since you have reviewed the guidelines and standards under which we practice, right? Unless you have been studying for a new license or certificate you are likely to be rusty on the ethical standards of our work.

So then I offer Chapter 3 to you as a good opportunity to brush up on the "Do's And Don'ts." The Ethical Standards of the American Psychological Association and the American Association of Marriage and Family Counselors are presented there. This review will help you scrutinize your present practice, and will help you to evaluate the many ideas and methods that you will find in this handbook.

Then feel free to combine, integrate, discard, modify, reverse, reject, or in any way apply any and all ideas presented herein. And in passing, may I encourage you to share them with me for future editions of this handbook?

Here's to your renewed and resoundingly successful practice!

To You, The Instructor

I was not fortunate enough to have a course available in the practical matters of setting up a private practice while slugging it out in grad school. But now things are different, I'm happy to say. More and more counseling and psychology programs are offering some formal course work related to the business of independent practice. And the classes are always full.

As I mentioned to the newcomers, a heavy emphasis should be placed on those chapters dealing with readiness for ones own practice, and the risks inherent in the activity, the "how to's" of fading into one's own practice, and, of course, the ethical guidelines that are fundamental to the work. Therefore, in any formal class time spent in preparation for independent practice, licensing, etc. the greater balance of time might be well spent in Chapters 1 through 3 inclusive. Chapter 10 offers some of the daily "headache" or maintenance chores that are important for the novice to note — since private work is anything but a rose garden (there are also the thorns!).

In addition to the material offered here, may I suggest another adjunct activity that would greatly benefit the student? Perhaps the student with no experience whatever could consult with experienced therapists in the community regarding the pluses and minuses of the business of private practice. I have received such calls myself and am always glad to give time over the phone to advise the sincere student.

And in your work with those fresh, creative minds of your students, I would also encourage you to share new ideas and approaches with future readers of this handbook by dropping me a line. Due credit for publication will be acknowledged with thanks.

And finally, **TO YOU**, whatever your tenure or position, one last remark. The hundreds of ideas and plans and wild notions in this book are not all of my own invention. I have borrowed ideas liberally from too many sources to catalogue here — sources to whom I am sincerely grateful. The discovery of these techniques and their power in building a successful practice has been thrilling.

But there is one more discovery that I made in the journey to a fuller and more meaningful life through private practice. That incredible discovery you will find described in Chapter 12.

We cannot achieve a better income, become better therapists, or manage a better private practice unless we first learn how to live better lives. When you reach Chapter 12 you will discover, as I did, the greatest "secret" of all.

Charles H. Browning
January, 1979

TABLE OF CONTENTS

*See page 234
for important information . . .*

LIST OF FIGURES

PRIVATE
PRACTICE
HANDBOOK

INTRODUCTION

INTRODUCTION

This Handbook and the success of our own private practice owe much to the creative nagging of my wife, Bev. Of course, she would not call it nagging. Her definition for the activity goes something like this: "gently helping me to see things in the proper perspective." Anyway, during one of those slow, no-patients-scheduled afternoons while I was relaxing with a book, Bev turned to me and said, "Honey, don't you really think that you're treating this practice like a hobby?" "Like a *hobby!*" I defensively responded, "Of course not!" I launched into a string of rational and logical excuses to justify the meager growth of our practice to that date, and failed to see the "proper perspective."

It was only after I had exhausted all my alibis that I could face the truth. Having a successful private practice had been a dream of mine for years. I had engaged in all phases of fantasy about that activity from the time I was a Junior in the university. And when the day finally arrived when I set up the practice *in vivo,* I had made a serious blunder. Somehow in the midst of my dreaming I had the expectation that when I got an office, printed business cards, and hired an answering service that patients would flock to the door. But they didn't come . . . not even in small groups, much less flocks! Indeed I was treating the practice as a hobby! For my dream to become a reality I had to put aside dreaming and playing at the business of a professional practice and conduct the practice as a professional business activity.

But clinicians typically do not like to think of themselves as "in business" even from a professional point of view. And it wasn't until I overcame this aversion that our own practice began to thrive. A professional private practice in the final analysis is a *professional business endeavor.*

Someone has rightly said that the success of any business venture results when our thinking, imagination, efforts, and our actions are organized into a definite pattern and are directed toward a specific goal and are pursued with untiring and enthusiastic energy. The professional private practice is no exception. For a private practice to grow and reach the point in which you are in a position to rely on it as your sole source of income to support your family comfortably, you must accept the fact that you are a professional businessman or woman. You must also resign yourself to living a business-like life and broadening your skills beyond the clinical arena. Most of us as therapists have had the luxury in the hospital or clinic or university milieu of having someone else handle the administrative and planning phases of our work. But now *you* become the administrator, the bookkeeper, the coffee maker, the practice developer, as well as the therapist.

The business of developing a successful private practice is not unlike raising your own precious child. During the early stages of growth the child is totally helpless and dependent on you. You must mobilize all available resources to care for his needs. You must get up in the middle of the night to feed him. But as he grows he is able to do more and more on his own and to sustain himself.

In the early going you must invest much time and organized planning to "feed" your practice. This involves the utilization of certain principles of organization and systematic planning to introduce yourself and your work to your community and to other professionals. By creative and careful implementation of certain techniques and methods in an orderly manner, your practice will develop rapidly and healthily. And like the little child who eventually can walk on his own, with the *consistent* application of organized planning in the early phases, your practice will be sustained in later phases by word-of-mouth referrals.

The principles and ideas outlined in this handbook represent the results of much trial-and-error learning, much of it accumulated by us (with many gray hairs in the process), and much of it borrowed from other successful practices. It is our sincere hope that whether you are just beginning your own practice, or whether you are preparing to expand your practice, that we can save you your own gray hairs and point the way to a smoother growth for your practice. Ultimately and most importantly, if the suggestions in this manual help you broaden your outreach to your community, many more patients will be served and lives changed for the better.

In this manual you will learn how to apply many business-oriented principles to the management of your own practice in an orderly way. And we are aware that this orientation may offend the clinical consciences of some. To those we simply ask for your patient understanding and open-mindedness. Read through the handbook. And as you would do with a menu in a fine restaurant, select only those specialties that appeal to your personal taste, leaving the rest for others.

Finally, let us offer two suggestions for your consideration of this material. (1) As you encounter an idea that is perhaps new to your thinking, before you reject it as silly or impractical, spend some time using your creative imagination. Try to picture in your mind actually putting the idea into operation yourself. Project yourself into the method and consider the possible outcomes for your practice and in your specific community. Someone once said, "Don't knock apples if you've never bitten into one." You just may be surprised at the power of an idea that at first glance seemed silly!

(2) Although it is important to conduct the successful practice in accordance with laws of order, organization and business know-how, as professional therapists our first responsibility is to our professional ethical standards. Without ethical standards we simply do what feels right, and feelings are fickle things. Therefore, take every method or idea suggested in this manual, and those variations that you develop, and lay them side by side with the ethical standards of your professional organization. If there is even the slightest doubt in your mind as to the conformity of that method, discard it altogether. In the long run, an independent practice can only succeed to the extent that it reflects the highest standards of conduct.

If you can accept the fact that to be in private practice is to be in business, a professional business; and if you can commit yourself to abide by the strictest ethical guidelines, then the ideas and principles which you are about to explore will fascinate and intrigue you. But remember: *Success is truth acted upon.* As you read, use the manual like you would a cookbook. Read to apply! *Do* what you read. We are preparing this manual not just to sell books, but to share with you some ideas that result in thriving professional private practices. But the ideas only produce results when someone ACTS upon them!

As you encounter each idea or strategy, ask yourself these questions: "How can I implement this idea in this community? When can I schedule the time soon to put it into operation? What would be the best order to go about it here in this community? What do the Ethical Standards of my group say about such an idea? Do I have the necessary licenses, permits, experience, facilities and capital to successfully carry out this plan? — and if not, how can I get them?"

With this clearly in mind, let's consider now whether private practice is for *you,* and if you are for private practice.

CHAPTER ONE

TO BE OR NOT TO BE
IN PRIVATE PRACTICE

CHAPTER I
TO BE OR NOT TO BE
IN PRIVATE PRACTICE

Before the marriage there must be compatibility. The partners must be well suited to one another before plans are considered for a wedding. Are you compatible to a private practice of your own? Is she suitable and complimentary to you and to your personality? Before you make the decision to launch out in your own practice, or before you decide to significantly expand your present work in an independent practice, pause here and get to know each other better. Invest some time in a careful examination of some of the parameters of your decision to enter private practice or expand it. That decision will certainly have a profound impact on your life.

The following considerations are designed to help you make the decision "To Be or Not To Be in Private Practice." These points will be especially valuable to you if you are considering a full-time practice either now or in the future. Let's take a look together at both sides, the positive side of your own practice, and the not-so-sunny side of the issue. Consider all the data, weigh the pluses and minuses; then decide.

What are the advantages of a private practice of your own?

(1) In your own practice you enjoy the freedom to direct the practice in your own way (within ethical limits), on your terms, and during hours that YOU select.

(2) You work in an office milieu that you choose and can design to suit your own taste, and in a location that meets your needs best.

(3) You work with patients and colleagues with whom you work most effectively (no one is arbitrarily assigned to you — you screen all potential patients).

(4) You determine how and how much you are to be paid (in line with rates of other professionals in your area).

(5) You supervise those therapists whom you choose, and you decide when, how, and for how long to supervise them.

(6) In private practice you have the luxury of maximal flexibility: Your clinical work can more readily reflect your personality, style, beliefs and attitudes. You are more free to experiment with innovative techniques and methods.

(7) You ARE the boss! There is no one looking over your shoulder. But of course, none of us ever outgrow the need for good supervision, or at least sensitive and constructive feedback from colleagues.

(8) You are freed from the web of the bureaucracy! The only red tape, forms, reports, scheduling nightmares, and administrative gymnastics that you will encounter are those which YOU instigate. And you will. You will be surprised to discover that after a short time you will by necessity begin to create your own little bureaucracy of sorts. You are now the clinician *and* the administration! We will give you some tips for making this job a bit easier in Chapters 9 and 10.

(9) You are free to conduct research of your own choosing. And if you are patient and tough enough to withstand the rewrites, published papers in reputable journals is an excellent way to increase referrals from professionals. However, we are realistic enough to know that this point will not excite too many of you, since clinicians tend to be somewhat less than prolific in this area (and unfortunately I speak from experience!).

(10) You are fortunate enough in private practice to have the opportunity to initiate an enterprise from ground zero, and through your own creative energy and skill, watch it grow and develop into the fulfillment of your professional and financial dreams; a dream come true! And believe me, it is a special thrill and an exhilarating experience that will enrich your life.

(11) You are the decision-and-policy-maker in all aspects of your work.

(12) In private practice you have a ready-made barometer of your professional competence and effectiveness — the number of patients listed in your weekly appointment book, the number of successful terminations, the rate of patient referrals from the community and from colleagues, and the number of word-of-mouth referrals give you clear-cut data to assess your own performance and those who you supervise. This is accountability at its best!

(13) Private practice seems to act as a sort of special motivator. Because you rely on the practice for your total or major source of income, you are reminded of your own responsibility to "go the extra mile" for your patients and with the community, to keep up with professional literature and to update your repertoire of skills. Private practice keeps you on your toes professionally.

(14) And last, but certainly not "least," your own practice offers you a potential income far above the norm. Less than 8% of the population of the United States is engaged in self-employment, and the highest income levels are among this group. The limits on your income in private practice in almost any city are limited only by your professional competence, your creative imagination, your energy level, your ability to accept the uncertainties and take the risks in the activity, and by *those limitations that you place on yourself.* The methods and suggestions offered in this manual are intended to help you stimulate your creative planning and to remove those limitations.

If you think that the advantages outlined above only scratch the surface of the potential in a private practice of your own, you're right!

What are the disadvantages of a private practice?

Someone wisely remarked, "every refuge has its price." This is true of private practice. Before you make that final decision to begin or expand your practice, take advantage of the experience and reports of the "seasoned" therapists who can show you the other side of the matter. Just for a moment, then, let's look at the "price" you can expect to pay for choosing the private practice route.

(1) In a private practice *you are* the administration. Until you hire secretarial help, all the red-tape nuts and bolts rest firmly and heavily on your shoulders. Perhaps for the first time you are responsible for paying the rent, maintaining a business phone and answering service, handling insurance billing, purchasing office supplies and equipment, *ad infinitum.* After a short while in your own practice you will develop a new appreciation for those administrators that you used to take for granted!

(2) In your own practice you will become acutely aware of what the words *"progressive* income tax" really mean, especially around April fifteenth! You now must set aside enough money yourself to cover both State and Federal taxes, and pay what is called the "estimated taxes" quarterly. Plan to enlist the services of a good C.P.A. if you plan full- or even part-time practice. Because when you open your office you have a silent partner; his name is Uncle Sam!

(3) Moving into your own practice typically requires a considerable outlay of cash. There's the rent (first and last month),

phone, answering service, stationery, business cards, office signs, bank accounts and countless other "little things." And there are no guarantees as to the number of patients who will find their way to your waiting room, or when they will come. So you must be ready and willing to accept a certain amount of uncertainty and risk financially, at least in the early going. We will talk more about this later.

(4) There are times when you'll be lonely. Many therapists who move into private practice have come from clinics or hospitals or university counseling centers. Private practice does not offer the same opportunities for socializing or brainstorming with colleagues as do other settings. You may spend hours and hours seeing patients or taking care of paper work without any interaction with colleagues. Prepare for some lonesome time.

(5) You are now personally responsible for the success or failure of this enterprise. *You* must reach out and let the community know you exist. *You* are your own public relations man! Clinicians typically do not care for this role, but you must accept it nevertheless. We'll show you some ways to handle this in a systematic and ethical manner later.

(6) Practicing on your own, you are no longer covered by the agency's professional liability insurance coverage. It is a MUST to purchase your own professional malpractice insurance, even should you see only one patient per week. I have never personally known anyone who has been accused of malpractice in private practice, but you cannot rely on their good fortune. Without good insurance you leave your family and all you possess vulnerable. The most inexpensive means of purchasing liability insurance is through your professional association.

(7) To succeed in private practice you must be a self-starter, score high in self-discipline and self-confidence, and function well without much structure or direction. You are the captain of the ship, you plot the course, and you man the controls. If you are the type who requires a great deal of structure as to when, where, with whom, for how long and what to do from an external source, you'll find private practice uncomfortable at best, and frightening to behold! Many times you can tell a lot about the success one will have in private practice by his performance on independent study

courses while in school, and during his thesis or dissertation work. Think back on your own behavior during those unstructured times.

(8) You will doubtless require the services of a telephone answering service in the early going, at least until you hire a full-time secretary. This will prove to be a good test of your patience, endurance, and your empathic understanding! And should you manage to find a service that treats your patients with gentleness and kindness and that correctly takes down the callers' numbers, please let me know!

(9) If you elect to use a monthly billing system for the collection of patient fees, you face the uncomfortable situation of unpaid bills and how to collect them. Credit and collection agencies are one solution, but it is a messy and, in my opinion, a professionally unnecessary approach. After all, we are here to alleviate human suffering, not to add to it. The pay-as-you-go approach is much to be preferred (more about this in Chapter 9).

(10) Free time to "play" or be with your family may become a rare thing. We have had to adjust to eating dinner at 9 or 10 p.m.! And after a while you may have to search your dictionary for the meaning of the word, "vacation."

(11) Until your practice reaches a self-sustaining level, you can expect that your patience, confidence, and your frustration tolerance level will be put to the test. Prepare for the "roller coaster effect!"

The Roller Coaster Effect

After working in a clinic, hospital or counseling center for some time one becomes a bit complacent with regard to patient flow. In most settings that have been established for a while there seems to be a steady stream of those in need of your services. There may even be a waiting list.

But in the early going on your own you don't have such a luxury. Most therapists report that in the early phases of a private practice the number of patients that are entered in their appointment book fluctuates dramatically. We call this phenomenon the "Roller Coaster Effect."

Let's take a typical example of a therapist who has entered into his own practice and it has been functioning for about two months. Through referrals from a colleague and a local hospital, he has built his patient load up to seven patients seen weekly. His fee is $50 per hour. This works out to a gross income of $350 per week, or $1,400 per month. For a multitude of reasons, suddenly in the space of two weeks his patient load drops to two scheduled appointments per week! Without warning his weekly gross income falls to $100 and his monthly receipts plummet to $400. As you can see, this makes for some unsettled moments when the mortgage comes due!

The etiology of the patient drop-off is multifaceted. Lack of motivation, resistance, financial pressures, fear, family resistance to therapy, impatience for results — all combine to keep patients from following through. On the therapist's side of the ledger — he or she may project some uneasiness at the early stages of his or her own practice and the patient perceives it; the therapist may feel uncomfortable and awkward in handling the issue of fees; and often the one with a new practice slips into "over-trying" and may rush things a bit in order to bring about desired results. And this only begins to tap the "why's" of the problem.

When Edison was experimenting with electricity and trying to produce light with it, he never assumed that there was any fault in the power of electricity when his experiment failed. He assumed total responsibility for the lack of success. He attributed the difficulty to something that *he* had or had not done in manipulating variables. In the operation of a private practice we must do the same thing if we are to reduce patient fall-out.

Whatever the reason may be on the side of the patient for his or her termination, we like to put that on the shelf and assume 100% of the responsibility ourselves for that termination. Why? Because should we attribute the reason for his absence to some factor in the patient, however valid it may sound, we are left without any means by which to control for it. On the other hand should the therapist accept full responsibility, (i.e., attribute patient's absence entirely to something he did or didn't do, did or didn't say), then the therapist can modify his own behavior and reduce the fall-out tomorrow. Yes, the patient shares the burden. But we are interested here in keeping patients working on their difficulties and finding answers, and keeping the practice healthy. We will deal more at length with the "100% responsibility rule" later (see p. 151), but for now, suffice it to say that YOU are the one who determines the ups and downs of the roller coaster. YOU control its speed. And ultimately YOU will be credited with its leveling off and stabilizing! For now however, be advised; prepare for the roller coaster effect.

Before leaving this subject of caution, let me share a word of encouragement. After your practice reaches a certain level and once you have begun to implement certain strategies of practice development (such as those offered in the following pages) the dips become more gentle and predictable. In our own experience, we found that once we reached a caseload of approximately twenty patients per week the roller coaster leveled off and the practice rose steadily from that figure. Many colleagues confirm this finding in their own practices.

As you prepare to make any change in your present job, or to purchase office space, or hire additional staff, consider the roller coaster effect. Take care, but remember — it is an exhilarating ride, and it's better to have ridden it through, plunging and soaring, than never to have ridden it at all!

To Be Or Not To Be?

As your guide, I have touched briefly on some of the signposts that the experienced traveler along this way has learned the hard way. Now before continuing the journey into the nuts-and-bolts of practice development, pause here with me and ask yourself some searching questions. Especially if you are just contemplating starting a practice, ask yourself these questions to better understand the demands that a private practice makes on your life and whether this is the way you wish to travel.

Professional Readiness

	YES	NO
(1) Do I now possess the professional competence and skills necessary to render mental health services on an independent basis?	☐	☐
(2) Am I duly licensed and qualified to practice in this state and county?	☐	☐
(3) Is there some more experienced or knowledgeable therapist whom I respect who would be willing to supervise or provide feedback to my private work?	☐	☐

18

(4) In the past, has my work with patients indicated that:

    a) rapid and lasting change result from my intervention? ☐ ☐

    b) the incidence of suicide attempts, threats, and emergency psychiatric hospitalization has been rare among my patients? ☐ ☐

    c) the rate of early or premature termination from therapy has been extremely low among my patients? ☐ ☐

(5) Can I obtain Professional Liability Insurance to protect me and my family while engaged in private practice? ☐ ☐

Personal Readiness

                                                  YES   NO

(1) An independent practice of my own demands many hours per week in practice promotions and sessions with patients. Will my family accept and support this investment of time and energy outside the home? Is my spouse enthusiastic about the idea? ☐ ☐

(2) Will my present employer approve of "moonlighting" in my own practice? ☐ ☐

(3) Knowing that I am far from an objective observer of myself, are there *any* personal problems or conflicts in my own life that need attention and resolution before I enter private practice? ☐ ☐

How would they affect my patients' progress?

(4) Will my health permit me to meet the demands of my own practice? ☐ ☐

(5) Do I realistically have the time now to devote to a private practice? ☐ ☐

(6) Do I function well in the midst of frustration, uncertainty, and risk taking? ☐ ☐

(7) Am I willing to accept infringement on my private/personal time taken up by phone calls from patients on evenings, weekends, and holidays? ☐ ☐

Readiness For Self-Employment

	YES	NO
(1) Am I willing to accept full responsibility for the success or failure of my own practice?	☐	☐
(2) Can I effectively organize my time, plan and work efficiently *without* structure?	☐	☐
(3) Do I have complete confidence and believe in my own ability to develop a successful practice?	☐	☐
(4) Am I willing to spend time in practice promotions, public relations and presentation making to tell my community and other professionals that I have a practice?	☐	☐
(5) Can I make and stick by my decisions?	☐	☐
(6) Can I comfortably handle the matter of collecting the fee directly from patients?	☐	☐
(7) Can I afford a potential change in my present tax bracket?	☐	☐
(8) Am I able to persevere and persist in the face of successive set-backs, failures and adversity?	☐	☐
(9) Am I willing to accept the many administrative duties (e.g., scheduling, fee collection, insurance billing, bill paying, supply purchasing, insurance coverage, licensing, etc.) and still maintain the highest level of professional performance?	☐	☐
(10) Am I willing to govern my practice, in all phases, according to the ethical standards of my profession?	☐	☐

If after careful and serious consideration of these questions you found yourself responding with several "NO" answers, you might do well at this time to postpone setting out on your own. Perhaps these questions suggested areas of your life in which you need special attention to prepare for your own practice.

If the scales are tipped in the "YES" direction, then let's begin our journey together, exploring ways to build and nourish a thriving, rewarding, and exciting practice of your own.

CHAPTER TWO

HOW TO SET UP THE PRACTICE

CHAPTER 2
HOW TO SET UP THE PRACTICE

The journey of a thousand miles
begins with but a single step

Once convinced of your suitability and overall readiness to enter your own practice, you are faced with a decision: "Where do I begin?"

You are establishing a practice to provide mental health services to your community. You begin by first determining whether there is a *need* for your services in the community — a need that you can satisfy. Once you determine the need, you must decide *where* you will see patients; where you will render your services. These matters must be wrestled with and settled even before you have your first prospective patient.

In this chapter we will discuss how to determine whether your city or town can utilize your services, and how to go about finding that first office.

Is There A Sufficient Need For Your Services?

Three psychologists met together for lunch during a national conference of their professional association. All three therapists were employed in hospital settings, and all were interested in "someday" launching out into their own private work. While waiting for their meal to arrive, the subject turned to the feasibility of setting up a practice in their home towns. It went something like this:

DR. A: "I would love to set up a practice in my city and break away from the hospital, but I don't think that the population of my community would support a full-time practice . . ."

DR. B: "Well, my situation is just reversed; the population of our city is growing by leaps and bounds. But in our area there must be 15 therapists per every square block! How could I compete against that kind of competition?"

DR. C: "I've put off trying my own practice in earnest because Jim Jones tried making a go of his own practice last year and he had to close up his office after only six months."

On the face of it, each argument seems to be valid, doesn't it? And in one sense they are. Population size, population/therapist ratios, and the track record of others are to be taken into account. But when we look a bit deeper at the needs that their special kind of services are designed to meet, we see something most interesting. Namely this: Unlike other business enterprises, either offering services or products, the professional business of psychotherapy has a potential clientele as large as the community itself! Why? How many people do you know who have *no* areas of conflict, frustration or troublesome habit pattern in their lives? The demand for your services is universal in your community because your services are directed at bringing about peace of mind, harmonious relationships, and meaningful living. If one is awake and breathing he is a potential patient!

What about therapist density? If there were indeed 15 therapists per block, would this contraindicate the decision to begin a practice? Answer this question by considering how a patient finds a therapist. If a potential patient walked up and down each block knocking on doors comparing therapists then this argument might hold up. But do they do that? Of course not. They are *referred* to the therapist by someone who knows of the therapist's work — a doctor, a friend, a co-worker, a pastor or priest, a hot line, etc. Therapist density is therefore irrelevant, even in Beverly Hills, California! Similarly, the success or failure of Jim Jones is an unreliable measure of the potential for a practice. Jim Jones may not have been suited to that community — but you may be.

In nearly every community today the need is overwhelming. Glance through your morning paper tomorrow to see the suffering and pain in your neighborhood. The real issue is that most clinicians have never been trained in the fine art of how to tell their neighbors that they can help them. We call this process "practice development." You will be guided step-by-step in the how-to's of introducing yourself to your community in later sections of this handbook.

Someone has accurately said that "success does not require reasons, only *results*."

When To Begin Your Own Practice?

A builder does not wait until he has a sure buyer before he constructs a home. General Motors does not hold off making a Cadillac until they have a buyer. Why? Because they know that the need for their product exists. The need in your community for peace of mind is equal to that of shelter and transportation. So, if you have examined the material in Chapter One with care, and still believe that the way of private practice is for you, BEGIN NOW!

Unlike most business or professional activities, you need almost no inventory, equipment or supplies. You require simply an appropriate place for you and the patient to sit down and converse. You can begin a practice with practically *no* outlay of cash whatever!

Can Your Home Also Be Your Office?

You have two choices open to you. You can set up your office in your own home, or you can move into a professional office building. Which is best? We come against a controversial issue here among our colleagues. I do not pretend to have the "final answer" on the matter, but rather than sidestep the question, I will offer my *opinion* outright — and it is only that.

Seeing patients out of your own home has some definite advantages to be sure. You incur no additional monthly rent expense. There is no necessity for an added telephone installation. You eliminate transportation and parking expenses. You gain more time with your family. And there is a certain informality about it that some therapists feel puts the patient more at ease.

With all the "pluses" of the home-office, I must express my personal preference, and my recommendation to you, in favor of the professional-office. Why? If your office is in your own home, you significantly reduce the potential for referrals from other professionals in your area. This is especially true for those patients referred by physicians. And of course, in building a practice you want to do everything ethically possible to *increase* referral potential!

Maintaining the office in your home dramatically reduces the climate of privacy for you and your family — and in our profession, we need as much quality alone-time with our family as possible. In addition, your privacy with patients may be affected by distractions from the kids or just normal household activities.

So my bias is clear. But to help *you* decide where to begin your own practice, consider this question carefully, then decide.

QUESTION: "Name all the professional people you know, or know of, who practice out of their own homes: Other therapists? Physicians? Attorneys? Dentists? C.P.A.'s?, etc?" Your own answer to this question should help you decide the most appropriate place to practice your *profession*.

The Sink-Or-Swim Approach to Private Practice

One well-known east coast therapist recommends that the newcomer to private practice make up his mind to "sink or swim." He suggests that the therapist, with or without previous experience in private practice, decide on the community that he wishes to live in, do some research on the area, quit his job, take out a loan for $20,000, and jump in with wild abandon.

The assumption apparently is that when one burns his boats and bridges behind him, he is much more likely to succeed due to survival motivation. There is something to be said for this in principle, and it works with some courageous souls. But is it for you? If the only way you function well is under threat of disaster perhaps this is the approach of choice.

But those of us who are not so adventuresome might do better dipping a toe in, and then an ankle, and then up to the knee, and so forth. I recommend to prospective practitioners that they use the process or "Fade-In" method of setting up shop.

How To Gently "Fade In" To Your Own Practice

The Fade–In, or step-by-step process approach to beginning a practice offers many advantages to the newcomer who is neither famous in his community nor independently wealthy. Using this avenue of building a practice you are not required to foot the bill of your own office or furnish it right away; which runs into a bundle of money! The Fade-In method takes advantage of the already existing facilities of others and allows you to begin seeing patients with the minimal risk financially to you.

How does this approach work in practice? It's simple. Rather than setting up your own office, *begin by subletting office space*. Let's consider some practical guidelines for subletting.

Guidelines For Subletting Office Space

What does it mean to "sublet"? To avoid risking your own capital in the early phases of your practice, you simply find someone who already has office space of their own which is suitable for your work. You arrange with him to rent an office in his suite and agree to pay him a flat fee or a percentage of the fee you charge your patients. He bears the burden of all the office expenses while you pay rent for only that time you use the office. The benefit to you is obvious, at least in the early going. When you reach a certain level of patient hours you will want to move into your own office. But that bridge isn't upon us at this point.

Is Location Important? Many times a potential patient will choose *you* as their therapist based on your location, believe it or not. In the search for your office, be sure that the building is near the major population area of your city, is on a public transportation route, and is located in a respectable area. In California where we are addicted to freeway life, we recommend that the office be as near as possible to freeway access.

How to find someone to sublet to you. Once you have researched the area and have decided on where you would like to practice, you must find that friendly colleague with the empty chairs! A direct referral seems to be the most effective means to land the office space. For this reason it is wise to ask those whom you know in the field if they can recommend anyone who has office space in this area, and who might be willing to sublet. The "I was referred by So and So" is a good ice-breaker and helps your own credibility.

Should you have no success finding someone who knows someone, then you begin the process of hunting and pecking. Call the local professional association in your state or county and get their directory. Before calling their members in your area, don't forget to ask the secretary there if she can recommend someone. Secretaries often prove to be a storehouse of information. Call those members in the directory who are engaged in your particular specialty; e.g., psychology, marriage counseling, clinical social work, etc. Let them know that you were referred to them by the professional association, and that you too are a member (if this is the case). This helps to build rapport and camaraderie, and opens doors! If no luck with those in your specialty area, then call those who have offices that are equally equipped for therapy and ask if they have space to sublet.

If you still are empty handed, dig out the local Yellow Pages and follow the same procedure. Don't overlook the several possible headings: e.g., Psychologists, Marriage & Family Counselors, Psychiatrists, Alcoholism Treatment and Drug Centers, Social Workers, Clinics, etc.

Consider everyone whom you call a potential lead to just the right person. Should they have no space themselves, *always* ask this question before hanging up; "I really do appreciate your time. Would you happen to know of someone who might be interested in subletting some unused office space?" This has several advantages to you: (1) you increase the probability of finding someone; (2) you shorten the hunt; and (3) you may end up with a direct referral!

Finding suitable office space for your work is really not much of a problem. Remember, it is to his advantage to let space to you — while he is working with a patient, or even on the golf course, his office is earning money. Everybody wins in subletting.

Key questions to ask before subletting. You have found someone who is eager to sublet to you. You get together to talk it over and *you* are the buyer, so ask some precision questions that will help you decide whether to use his space or look elsewhere. Get specific answers to the following questions:

"What are the parking arrangements for me, and for patients?"
"How near is the office to public transportation?"
"Is the office accessible for wheel chair patients?"
"How many offices are in the suite?"
"How many patients will the waiting room accommodate?"
"How late does the building stay open in the evenings, on holidays, on the weekends?"
"Are there any charges to me for having my name put on the door sign, the floor and central register of the building?"

(NOTE: Be sure to get agreement on these matters, because some landlords will permit only the tenant himself to display his sign and name. Having your own sign is a "must" for your practice! And it's expensive, so brace yourself!).

How to negotiate the rent. There are essentially two methods commonly used in determining how much you will pay for the use of office space: (1) a flat hourly rate, versus (2) a rate based on percentage-of-fee-income. Let's examine them both.

—*The Flat Hourly Rate.* A specific charge is made for each hour you occupy the office, regardless of what you charge your patients. The typical rate these days in Southern California is somewhere between $7 and $15 per hour. The main advantage to you under this system is that in the long run you pay less for office space if your fees are in parity with the going rate. Also, if you plan to run groups, this is the preferred arrangement. But be careful! Many tenants offer this method and charge you for the hours you actually *schedule* the space, whether your patient shows up or not, and regardless of whether they pay you or not! You can readily see the risk here — if the patient doesn't show up or fails to pay for services, you are out $7-$15. If this method is proposed to you, get him to agree that you pay the flat fee *only* if the patient keeps the scheduled appointment. If he rejects this arrangement, propose to him the percentage method.

—*The Percentage-Of-Fee-Income Method.* Under the percentage approach, you agree to pay the tenant a specified percentage or proportion of all monies that you take in from patient fees. The going rate in Southern California is from 20% to 60%. This is paid on a weekly or monthly basis. For example, let's say you see five patients per week @ $50 per hour under a 25% percentage arrangement. At the end of one month your rent is $250.00 (25% of $1,000). For a contrast, under the flat rate method considering the same patient hours, at a $10 hourly rate your rent would be $200 (20 hrs. X $10). The obvious advantages of the percentage arrangement are that you pay rent only on actual money taken in; you are not penalized for no-shows, cancellations, those who fail to pay on time, or for insurance payments which sometimes take forever.

A friendly word of advice: If the tenant proposes a flat rate significantly above $15 per hour, or a percentage in excess of 40%, I suggest you look elsewhere. Also, you may be offered an hourly wage if you will see patients that he refers to you through his practice. This is a tempting arrangement especially if you are just starting out, but resist it! Remember, your ultimate objective is a thriving and self-sustaining practice *of your own.* Working for the tenant may give security, but you will never experience the thrill of developing your own practice, and you lose autonomy to implement the methods in this manual for yourself. Keep your respective practices distinct and separate.

To summarize: The flat hourly rate is preferable if you have very few patients and if you charge below the going rate, and if tenant will charge only for time patients are actually seen. The percentage-of-fee-income is preferable if you charge the going rate, have many patients who defer payment for whatever reason, and the rate is reasonable. Finally, remain a subletter, not an employee!

Assess Space and Time Availability. Many tenants sublet their office space to several subletters. Before you decide to move in, check out the total number of open hours available to you during times that you can see patients. If the office suite seems a bit crowded now, you can be sure that you will run into scheduling conflicts later. You would want to get some assurance that certain blocks of time would be made available for you when needed.

Have Your Own Designated Office. We have heard horror stories (and lived through one ourselves!) in which the subletter arrived to see his patients and found himself shuffled about from one room to another to accommodate other therapists who happened to have more seniority in that office. The effect on both therapist and patient was less than desirable, to put it mildly. So from the very outset get an agreement that you will work in *one* designated office only, when you are scheduled to use the suite, and that that office is adequately furnished.

Sharing the tenant's answering service. Ask the tenant if he will include your name on his answering service, or have his secretary take your messages. This is the customary arrangement and is covered under your rent payment at no additional charge. Ask him to inform the secretary or the service that you are now receiving messages in this office, and give them your home phone number for emergency calls, etc. He will give you his "code number" and the number of the answering service. Use the code number when you call in for your messages. While we are on the subject of answering services, it is a good idea to call your service once or more times daily, even in the early phases when you have no calls coming in. Why? Because the girls who work the board get to know you and they will give you more efficient service if they expect that you may be calling in periodically. We will have more to say in Chapter 9 with regard to the answering service.

What about telephone answering machines? Although some therapists employ the phone taping machines, we feel their problems outweigh their strengths. In the first place, most people feel somewhat awkward talking to a tape recorder. Many people get all flustered, self-conscious, hang up, or forget to leave their phone number! This is especially true if the patient is a bit suspicious and does not like being recorded. Secondly, a machine is unable to make important decisions to track you down in case of an emergency or other important call. The phone answering machine lacks that important human factor so necessary in our professional relationships with patients.

Now that you have found just the perfect office arrangement and have the keys in your hand, what's next? Before you can begin to provide services to your community and inform them of your new practice, you must be absolutely certain that you understand and are willing to abide by the "rules of the game." Let's take time now in Chapter 3 to carefully consider the "rules" or ethical standards in private practice.

CHAPTER THREE

THE DO'S AND DON'TS
OF A SUCCESSFUL PROFESSIONAL PRACTICE

CHAPTER 3
THE DO'S AND DON'TS
OF A SUCCESSFUL PROFESSIONAL PRACTICE

Some time ago we purchased a sandbox for our children. It was not assembled, but came in pieces to be assembled. Among the many bags of parts, screws, nuts, bolts, and what-have-you, there were detailed instructions for assembly. I gave the instructions a quick glance, and set them aside, saying smugly to myself, "Who needs instructions to put together something as basic as a sandbox?" . . . Four hours later . . . I was perplexed, frustrated, and not so smug when the "basic" sandbox still remained mostly unassembled! As usual, my wife asked the key question as she came out in the garage to see what had happened to me and the "basic" sandbox. She asked with tongue in cheek, "Honey, didn't it come with instructions?"

Had I patiently studied the instructions, the rules for correct assembly, the kids would have had the sandbox three and a half hours earlier, and much unnecessary aggravation could have been avoided.

I share this little story with you because it nicely illustrates a truth in the "correct assembly" and maintenance of a successful professional private practice. For any practice to flourish and grow, it must function according to instructions — or rules or standards. We call these instructions a "code of ethics" or standards of professional conduct.

Like the instructions with my sandbox, they seem at first glance somewhat tedious or boring. They may even be thought non-essential or "basic." You may be tempted, as I was, to skim over or skip altogether the ethical guidelines outlined in this chapter. But do not yield unto temptation! In addition to the success or failure of your practice, these guidelines and principles will have direct impact on your patients' lives, your community, your profession, and your own personal integrity and reputation.

Know, understand, apply and abide by the highest standards of professional excellence and your chances of building a private practice that enriches the community and your own life are much enhanced. Before going on to the "How-To's" of developing referrals, spend some time here in the instruction section. This will be time well spent!

A successful professional practice actually *thrives* on limits, constraints of conduct, and principles of order. There is the story of the little train who got sick and tired of being restrained and bound to his two tracks all the time. He just wanted to "do his own thing" and to be "free." On his two limiting tracks he always had to go one way. But he wanted to explore the wide-open spaces on his own. So one day he took matters into his own hands and jumped off his tracks to do his own thing and see the world. You can guess how far he got! He learned to his surprise that although the tracks were limiting and confining, he could only move along smoothly and rapidly without any bumps or bruises if he held fast to those limits. After he got back on his two little tracks, he learned to love them and stay firmly planted on them at all times!

Let's take a look together at the "tracks" of your own practice. They're limiting to be sure, but they certainly do make the journey smoother. I have selected those professional standards for psychologists and for marriage and family counselors as representative ethical guidelines. For the success of your practice, spend some time with them now.

THE AMERICAN PSYCHOLOGICAL ASSOCIATION ETHICAL STANDARDS OF PSYCHOLOGISTS[1]

The psychologist believes in the dignity and worth of the individual human being. He is committed to increasing man's understanding of himself and others. While pursuing this endeavor, he protects the welfare of any person who may seek his service or of any subject, human or animal, that may be the object of his study. He does not use his professional position or relationships, nor does he knowingly permit his own services to be used by others for purposes inconsistent with these values. While demanding for himself freedom of inquiry and communication, he accepts the responsibility this freedom confers: for competence where he claims it, for objectivity in the report of his findings, and for consideration of the best interests of his colleagues and of society.

---

1. Reprinted by permission of APA. Copyrighted by the American Psychological Association, Inc., January 1963. Reprinted (and edited) from the *American Psychologist*, January 1963, and as amended by the APA Council of Representatives in September 1965 and December 1972. NOTE: Consult APA for updated code of ethics.

Specific Principles

Principle 1. Responsibility. The psychologist,[2] committed to increasing man's understanding of man, places high value on objectivity and integrity, and maintains the highest standards in the services he offers.

a. As a scientist, the psychologist believes that society will be best served when he investigates where his judgment indicates investigation is needed; he plans his research in such a way as to minimize the possibility that his findings will be misleading; and he publishes full reports of his work, never discarding without explanation data which may modify the interpretation of results.

b. As a teacher, the psychologist recognizes his primary obligation to help others acquire knowledge and skill, and to maintain high standards of scholarship.

c. As a practitioner, the psychologist knows that he bears a heavy social responsibility because his work may touch intimately the lives of others.

Principle 2. Competence. The maintenance of high standards of professional competence is a responsibility shared by all psychologists, in the interest of the public and of the profession as a whole.

a. Psychologists discourage the practice of psychology by unqualified persons and assist the public in identifying psychologists competent to give dependable professional service. When a psychologist or a person identifying himself as a psychologist violates ethical standards, psychologists who know firsthand of such activities attempt to rectify the situation. When such a situation cannot be dealt with informally, it is called to the attention of the appropriate local, state, or national committee on professional ethics, standards, and practices.

b. Psychologists regarded as qualified for independent practice are those who (a) have been awarded a Diploma by the American Board of Examiners in Professional Psychology, or (b) have been licensed or certified by state examining boards, or (c) have been certified by voluntary boards established by state psychological associations. Psychologists who do not yet meet the qualifications recognized for independent practice should gain experience under qualified supervision.

c. The psychologist recognizes the boundaries of his competence and the limitations of his techniques and does not offer services or use techniques that fail to meet professional standards established in particular fields. The psychologist who engages in practice assists his client in obtaining professional help for all important aspects of his problem that fall outside the boundaries of his own competence. This principle requires, for example, that provision be made for the diagnosis and treatment of relevant medical problems and for referral to or consultation with other specialists.

d. The psychologist in clinical work recognizes that his effectiveness depends in good part upon his ability to maintain sound interpersonal relations, that temporary or more enduring aberrations in his own personality may interfere with this ability or distort his appraisals of others. Therefore he refrains from undertaking any activity in which his personal problems are likely to result in inferior professional services or harm to a client; or, if he is already engaged in such an activity when he becomes aware of his personal problems, he seeks competent professional assistance to determine whether he should continue or terminate his services to his client.

---

2. A student of psychology who assumes the role of psychologist shall be considered a psychologist for the purpose of this code of ethics.

Principle 3. Moral and Legal Standards. The psychologist in the practice of his profession shows sensible regard for the social codes and moral expectations of the community in which he works, recognizing that violations of accepted moral and legal standards on his part may involve his clients, students, or colleagues in damaging personal conflicts, and impugn his own name and the reputation of his profession.

Principle 4. Misrepresentation. The psychologist avoids misrepresentation of his own professional qualifications, affiliations, and purposes, and those of the institutions and organizations with which he is associated.

a. A psychologist does not claim either directly or by implication professional qualifications that differ from his actual qualifications, nor does he misrepresent his affiliation with any institution, organization, or individual, nor lead others to assume he has affiliations that he does not have. The psychologist is responsible for correcting others who misrepresent his professional qualifications or affiliations.

b. The psychologist does not misrepresent an institution or organization with which he is affiliated by ascribing to it characteristics that it does not have.

c. A psychologist does not use his affiliation with the American Psychological Association or its Divisions for purposes that are not consonant with the stated purposes of the Association.

d. A psychologist does not associate himself with or permit his name to be used in connection with any services or products in such a way as to misrepresent them, the degree of his responsibility for them, or the nature of his affiliation.

Principle 5. Public Statements. Modesty, scientific caution, and due regard for the limits of present knowledge characterize all statements of psychologists who supply information to the public, either directly or indirectly.

a. Psychologists who interpret the science of psychology or the services of psychologists to clients or to the general public have an obligation to report fairly and accurately. Exaggeration, sensationalism, superficiality, and other kinds of misrepresentation are avoided.

b. When information about psychological procedures and techniques is given, care is taken to indicate that they should be used only by persons adequately trained in their use.

c. A psychologist who engages in radio or television activities does not participate in commercial announcements recommending purchase or use of a product.

Principle 6. Confidentiality. Safeguarding information about an individual that has been obtained by the psychologist in the course of his teaching, practice, or investigation is a primary obligation of the psychologist. Such information is not communicated to others unless certain important conditions are met.

a. Information received in confidence is revealed only after most careful deliberation and when there is clear and imminent danger to an individual or to society, and then only to appropriate professional workers or public authorities.

b. Information obtained in clinical or consulting relationships, or evaluative data concerning children, students, employees, and others are discussed only for professional purposes and only with persons clearly concerned with the case. Written and oral reports should present only data germane to the purposes of the evaluation, every effort should be made to avoid undue invasion of privacy.

c. Clinical and other materials are used in classroom teaching and writing only when the identity of the persons involved is adequately disguised.

d. The confidentiality of professional communications about individuals is maintained. Only when the originator and other persons involved give their express permission is a confidential professional communication shown to the individual concerned. The psychologist is responsible for informing the client of the limits of the confidentiality.

e. Only after explicit permission has been granted is the identity of research subjects published. When data have been published without permission for identification, the psychologist assumes responsibility for adequately disguising their sources.

f. The psychologist makes provisions for the maintenance of confidentiality in the preservation and ultimate disposition of confidential records.

Principle 7. Client Welfare. The psychologist respects the integrity and protects the welfare of the person or group with whom he is working.

a. The psychologist in industry, education, and other situations in which conflicts of interest may arise among various parties, as between management and labor, or between the client and employer of the psychologist, defines for himself the nature and direction of his loyalties and responsibilities and keeps all parties concerned informed of these commitments.

b. When there is a conflict among professional workers, the psychologist is concerned primarily with the welfare of any client involved and only secondarily with the interest of his own professional group.

c. The psychologist attempts to terminate a clinical or consulting relationship when it is reasonably clear to the psychologist that the client is not benefiting from it.

d. The psychologist who asks that an individual reveal personal information in the course of interviewing, testing, or evaluation, or who allows such information to be divulged to him, does so only after making certain that the responsible person is fully aware of the purposes of the interview, testing, or evaluation and of the ways in which the information may be used.

e. In cases involving referral, the responsibility of the psychologist for the welfare of the client continues until this responsibility is assumed by the professional person to whom the client is referred or until the relationship with the psychologist making the referral has been terminated by mutual agreement. In situations where referral, consultation, or other changes in the conditions of the treatment are indicated and the client refuses referral, the psychologist carefully weighs the possible harm to the client, to himself, and to his profession that might ensue from continuing the relationship.

f. The psychologist who requires the taking of psychological tests for didactic, classification, or research purposes protects the examiners by insuring that the tests and test results are used in a professional manner.

g. When potentially disturbing subject matter is presented to students, it is discussed objectively, and efforts are made to handle constructively any difficulties that arise.

h. Care must be taken to insure an appropriate setting for clinical work to protect both client and psychologist from actual or imputed harm and the profession from censure.

i. In the use of accepted drugs for therapeutic purposes special care needs to be exercised by the psychologist to assure himself that the collaborating physician provides suitable safeguards for the client.

Principle 8. Client Relationship. The psychologist informs his prospective client of the important aspects of the potential relationship that might affect the client's decision to enter the relationship.

a. Aspects of the relationship likely to affect the client's decision include the recording of an interview, the use of interview material for training purposes, and observation of an interview by other persons.

b. When the client is not competent to evaluate the situation (as in the case of a child), the person responsible for the client is informed of the circumstances which may influence the relationship.

c. The psychologist does not normally enter into a professional relationship with members of his own family, intimate friends, close associates, or others whose welfare might be jeopardized by such a dual relationship.

Principle 9. Impersonal Services. Psychological services for the purpose of diagnosis, treatment, or personalized advice are provided only in the context of a professional relationship, and are not given by means of public lectures or demonstrations, newspaper or magazine articles, radio or television programs, mail, or similar media.

a. The preparation of personnel reports and recommendations based on test data secured solely by mail is unethical unless such appraisals are an integral part of a continuing client relationship with a company, as a result of which the consulting psychologist has intimate knowledge of the client's personnel situation and can be assured thereby that his written appraisals will be adequate to the purpose and will be properly interpreted by the client. These reports must not be embellished with such detailed analyses of the subject's personality traits as would be appropriate only after intensive interviews with the subject. The reports must not make specific recommendations as to employment or placement of the subject which go beyond the psychologist's knowledge of the job requirements of the company. The reports must not purport to eliminate the company's need to carry on such other regular employment or personnel practices as appraisal of the work history, checking of references, past performance in the company.

Principle 10. Announcement of Services. A psychologist adheres to professional rather than commercial standards in making known his availability for professional services.

a. A psychologist does not directly solicit clients for individual diagnosis or therapy.

b. Individual listings in telephone directories are limited to name, highest relevant degree, certification status, address, and telephone number. They may also include identification in a few words of the psychologist's major areas of practice; for example, child therapy, personnel selection, industrial psychology. Agency listings are equally modest.

c. Announcements of individual private practice are limited to a simple statement of the name, highest relevant degree, certification or diplomate status, address, telephone number, office hours, and a brief explanation of the types of services rendered. Announcements of agencies may list names of staff members with their qualifications. They conform in other particulars with the same standards as individual announcements, making certain that the true nature of the organization is apparent.

d. A psychologist or agency announcing nonclinical professional services may use brochures that are descriptive of services rendered but not evaluative. They may be sent to professional persons, schools, business firms, government agencies, and other similar organizations.

e. The use in a brochure of "testimonials from satisfied users" is unacceptable. The offer of a free trial of services is unacceptable if it operates to misrepresent in any way the nature or the efficacy of the services rendered by the psychologist. Claims that a psychologist has unique skills or unique devices not available to others in the profession are made only if the special efficacy of these unique skills or devices has been demonstrated by scientifically acceptable evidence.

f. The psychologist must not encourage (nor, within his power, even allow) a client to have exaggerated ideas as to the efficacy of services rendered. Claims made to clients about the efficacy of his services must not go beyond those which the psychologist would be willing to subject to professional scrutiny through publishing his results and his claims in a professional journal.

Principle 11. Interprofessional Relations. A psychologists acts with integrity in regard to colleagues in psychology and in other professions.

a. Each member of the Association cooperates with the duly constituted Committee on Scientific and Professional Ethics and Conduct in the performance of its duties by responding to inquiries with reasonable promptness and completeness. A member taking longer than 30 days to respond to such inquiries shall have the burden of demonstrating that he acted with "reasonable promptness."

b. A psychologist does not normally offer professional services to a person receiving psychological assistance from another professional worker except by agreement with the other worker or after the termination of the client's relationship with the other professional worker.

c. The welfare of clients and colleagues requires that psychologists in joint practice or corporate activities make an orderly and explicit arrangement regarding the conditions of their association and its possible termination. Psychologists who serve as employers of other psychologists have an obligation to make similar appropriate arrangements.

Principle 12. Remuneration. Financial arrangements in professional practice are in accord with professional standards that safeguard the best interest of the client and the profession.

a. In establishing rates for professional services, the psychologist considers carefully both the ability of the client to meet the financial burden and the charges made by other professional persons engaged in comparable work. He is willing to contribute a portion of his services to work for which he receives little or no financial return.

b. No commission or rebate or any other form of remuneration is given or received for referral of clients for professional services.

c. The psychologist in clinical or counseling practice does not use his relationships with clients to promote, for personal gain or the profit of an agency, commercial enterprise of any kind.

d. A psychologist does not accept a private fee or any other form of remuneration for professional work with a person who is entitled to his services through an institution or agency. The policies of a particular agency may make explicit provision for private work with its clients by members of its staff, and in such instances the client must be fully apprised of all policies affecting him.

Principle 13. Test Security. Psychological tests and other assessment devices, the value of which depends in part on the naivete of the subject, are not reproduced or described in popular publications in ways that might invalidate the techniques. Access to such devices is limited to persons with professional interests who will safeguard their use.

a. Sample items made up to resemble those of tests being discussed may be reproduced in popular articles and elsewhere, but scorable tests and actual test items are not reproduced except in professional publications.

b. The psychologist is responsible for the control of psychological tests and other devices and procedures used for instruction when their value might be damaged by revealing to the general public their specific contents or underlying principles.

Principle 14. Test Interpretation. Test scores, like test materials, are released only to persons who are qualified to interpret and use them properly.

a. Materials for reporting test scores to parents, or which are designed for self-appraisal purposes in schools, social agencies, or industry are closely supervised by qualified psychologists or counselors with provisions for referring and counseling individuals when needed.

b. Test results or other assessment data used for evaluation or classification are communicated to employers, relatives, or other appropriate persons in such a manner as to guard against misinterpretation or misuse. In the usual case, an interpretation of the test result rather than the score is communicated.

c. When test results are communicated directly to parents and students, they are accompanied by adequate interpretive aids or advice.

Principle 15. Test Publication. Psychological tests are offered for commercial publication only to publishers who present their tests in a professional way and distribute them only to qualified users.

a. A test manual, technical handbook, or other suitable report on the test is provided which describes the method of constructing and standardizing the test, and summarizes the validation research.

b. The populations for which the test has been developed and the purposes for which it is recommended are stated in the manual. Limitations upon the test's dependability, and aspects of its validity on which research is lacking or incomplete, are clearly stated. In particular, the manual contains a warning regarding interpretations likely to be made which have not yet been substantiated by research.

c. The catalog and manual indicate the training or professional qualifications required for sound interpretation of the test.

d. The test manual and supporting documents take into account the principles enunciated in the *Standards for Educational and Psychological Tests and Manuals.*

e. Test advertisements are factual and descriptive rather than emotional and persuasive.

Principle 16. Research Precautions. The psychologist assumes obligations for the welfare of his research subjects, both animal and human.

The decision to undertake research should rest upon a considered judgment by the individual psychologist about how best to contribute to psychological science and to human welfare. The responsible psychologist weighs alternative directions in which personal energies and resources might be invested. Having made the decision to conduct research, psychologists must carry out their investigations with respect for the people who participate and with concern for their dignity and welfare. The Principles that follow make explicit the investigator's ethical responsibilities toward participants over the course of research, from the initial decision to pursue a study to the steps necessary to protect the confidentiality of research data. These Principles should be interpreted in terms of the contexts provided in the complete document [3] offered as a supplement to these Principles.

a. In planning a study the investigator has the personal responsibility to make a careful evaluation of its ethical acceptability, taking into account these Principles for research with human beings. To the extent that this appraisal, weighing scientific and humane values, suggests a deviation from any Principle, the investigator incurs an increasingly serious obligation to seek ethical advice and to observe more stringent safeguards to protect the rights of the human research participants.

b. Responsibility for the establishment and maintenance of acceptable ethical practice in research always remains with the individual investigator. The investigator is also responsible for the ethical treatment of research participants by collaborators, assistants, students, and employees, all of whom, however, incur parallel obligations.

c. Ethical practice requires the investigator to inform the participant of all features of the research that reasonably might be expected to influence willingness to participate, and to explain all other aspects of the research about which the participant inquires. Failure to make full disclosure gives added emphasis to the investigator's abiding responsibility to protect the welfare and dignity of the research participant.

d. Openness and honesty are essential characteristics of the relationship between investigator and research participant. When the methodological requirements of a study necessitate concealment or deception, the investigator is required to ensure the participant's understanding of the reasons for this action and to restore the quality of the relationship with the investigator.

e. Ethical research practice requires the investigator to respect the individual's freedom to decline to participate in research or to discontinue participation at any time. The obligation to protect this freedom requires special vigilance when the investigator is in a position of power over the participant. The decision to limit this freedom gives added emphasis to the investigator's abiding responsibility to protect the participant's dignity and welfare.

---

3. *Ethical Principles in the Conduct of Research with Human Participants,* available upon request from the American Psychological Association.

f. Ethically acceptable research begins with the establishment of a clear and fair agreement between the investigator and the research participant that clarifies the responsibilities of each. The investigator has the obligation to honor all promises and commitments included in that agreement.

g. The ethical investigator protects participants from physical and mental discomfort, harm and danger. If the risk of such consequences exists, the investigator is required to inform the participant of that fact, secure consent before proceeding, and take all possible measures to minimize distress. A research procedure may not be used if it is likely to cause serious and lasting harm to participants.

h. After the data are collected, ethical practice requires the investigator to provide the participant with a full clarification of the nature of the study and to remove any misconceptions that may have arisen. Where scientific or humane values justify delaying or withholding information, the investigator acquires a special responsibility to assure that there are no damaging consequences for the participant.

i. Where research procedures may result in undesirable consequences for the participant, the investigator has the responsibility to detect and remove or correct these consequences, including, where relevant, long-term aftereffects.

j. Information obtained about the research participants during the course of an investigation is confidential. When the possibility exists that others may obtain access to such information, ethical research practice requires that this possibility, together with the plans for protecting confidentiality, be explained to the participants as a part of the procedure for obtaining informed consent.

k. A psychologist using animals in research adheres to the provisions of the Rules Regarding Animals, drawn up by the Committee on Precautions and Standards in Animal Experimentation and adopted by the American Psychological Association.

l. Investigations of human subjects using experimental drugs (for example: hallucinogenic, psychotomimetic, psychedelic, or similar substances) should be conducted only in such settings as clinics, hospitals, or research facilities maintaining appropriate safeguards for the subjects.

Principle 17. Publication Credit. Credit is assigned to those who have contributed to a publication, in proportion to their contribution, and only to these.

a. Major contributions of a professional character, made by several persons to a common project, are recognized by joint authorship. The experimenter or author who has made the principal contribution to a publication is identified as the first listed.

b. Minor contributions of a professional character, extensive clerical or similar nonprofessional assistance, and other minor contributions are acknowledged in footnotes or in an introductory statement.

c. Acknowledgment through specific citations is made for unpublished as well as published material that has directly influenced the research or writing.

d. A psychologist who compiles and edits for publication the contributions of others publishes the symposium or report under the title of the committee or symposium, with his own name appearing as chairman or editor among those of the other contributors or committee members.

Principle 18. Responsibility toward Organization. A psychologist respects the rights and reputation of the institute or organization with which he is associated.

a. Materials prepared by a psychologist as a part of his regular work under specific direction of his organization are the property of that organization. Such materials are released for use or publication by a psychologist in accordance with policies or authorization, assignment of credit, and related matters which have been established by his organization.

b. Other material resulting incidentally from activity supported by any agency, and for which the psychologist rightly assumes individual responsibility, is published with disclaimer for any responsibility on the part of the supporting agency.

Principle 19. Promotional Activities. The psychologist associated with the development or promotion of psychological devices, books, or other products offered for commercial sale is responsible for ensuring that such devices, books, or products are presented in a professional and factual way.

a. Claims regarding performance, benefits, or results are supported by scientifically acceptable evidence.

b. The psychologist does not use professional journals for the commercial exploitation of psychological products, and the psychologist-editor guards against such misuse.

c. The psychologist with a financial interest in the sale or use of a psychological product is sensitive to possible conflict of interest in his promotion of such products and avoids compromise of his professional responsibilities and objectives.

THE AMERICAN ASSOCIATION OF MARRIAGE AND FAMILY COUNSELORS CODE OF PROFESSIONAL ETHICS*

Preamble

Members of the AAMFC are professional counselors trained in dealing with marriage and family problems. They are conscious of their special skills and aware of their professional boundaries. They perform their professional duties on the highest levels of integrity and confidentiality and will not hesitate to recommend assistance from other professional disciplines when circumstances dictate. They are committed to protect the public against, and will not hesitate to expose, unethical, incompetent and dishonorable practices. To maintain these high standards of service, members of the AAMFC have imposed upon themselves the following rules of conduct and will earn highest public confidence.

SECTION I. CODE OF PERSONAL CONDUCT

1. A Counselor provides professional service to anyone regardless of race, religion, sex, political affiliation, social or economic status, or choice of lifestyle. When a

---

* Copyright The American Association of Marriage & Family Counselors. Reprinted by permission of AAMFC. Consult AAMFC for updated code of ethics.

Counselor cannot offer service for any reason, he or she will make a proper referral. Counselors are encouraged to devote a portion of their time to work for which there is little or no financial return.

2. A Counselor will not use his or her counseling relationship to further personal, religious, political, or business interests.

3. A Counselor will neither offer nor accept payment for referrals, and will actively seek all significant information from the source of referral.

4. A Counselor will not knowingly offer service to a client who is in treatment with another counseling professional without consultation among the parties involved.

5. A Counselor will not disparage the qualifications of any colleague.

6. Every member of the AAMFC has an obligation to continuing education and professional growth in all possible ways, including active participation in the meetings and affairs of the Association.

7. A Counselor will not attempt to diagnose, prescribe for, treat or advise on problems outside the recognized boundaries of the Counselor's competence.

8. The Association encourages its members to affiliate with professional groups, clinics or agencies operating in the field of marriage and family life. Similarly, interdisciplinary contact and cooperation are encouraged.

SECTION II. RELATIONS WITH CLIENTS

1. A Counselor, while offering dignified and reasonable support, is cautious in prognosis and will not exaggerate the efficacy of his or her service.

2. The Counselor recognizes the importance of clear understandings on financial matters with his or her clients. Arrangements for payments are settled at the beginning of a counseling relationship.

3. A Counselor keeps records of each case, and stores them in such a way as to insure safety and confidentiality, in accordance with the highest professional and legal standards.

a. Information shall be revealed only to professional persons concerned with the case. Written and oral reports should present only data germane to the purposes of the inquiry; every effort should be made to avoid undue invasion of privacy.

b. The Counselor is responsible for informing the client of the limits of confidentiality.

c. Written permission shall be granted by the clients involved before data may be divulged.

d. Information is not communicated to others without consent of the client unless there is clear and immediate danger to an individual or to society, and then only to the appropriate family members, professional workers or public authorities.

4. A Counselor deals with relationships at varying stages of their history. While respecting at all times the clients' right to make their own decision, the Counselor has a duty to assess the situation according to the highest professional standards. In all circumstances, the Counselor will clearly advise a client that the decision to separate or divorce is the responsibility solely of the client. In such an event, the Counselor has the continuing responsibility to offer support and counsel during the period of readjustment.

SECTION III. RESEARCH AND PUBLICATION

1. The Counselor is obligated to protect the welfare of his or her research subjects. The conditions of the Human Subjects Experimentation shall prevail, as specified by the Department of Health, Education and Welfare guidelines.

2. Publication credit is assigned to those who have contributed to a publication, in proportion to their contribution, and in accordance with customary publication practices.

SECTION IV. IMPLEMENTATION

1. In accepting membership in the Association, each member binds himself or herself to accept the judgment of his or her fellow members as to standards of professional ethics, subject to the safeguards provided in this section. Acceptance of membership implies consent to abide by the acts of discipline herein set forth and as enumerated in the Bylaws of the Association. It is the duty of each member to safeguard these standards of ethical practice. Should a fellow member appear to violate this Code he or she may be cautioned through friendly remonstrance, colleague consultation with the party in question, or formal complaint may be filed in accordance with the following procedure:

a. Complaint of unethical practice shall be made in writing to the Chairperson of the Standing Committee on Ethics and Professional Practices and to the Executive Director. A copy of the complaint shall be furnished to the person or persons against whom it is directed.

b. Should the Standing Committee decide the complaint warrants investigation, it shall so notify the charged party(ies) in writing. When investigation is indicated, the Standing Committee shall constitute itself an Investigating Committee and shall include in its membership at least one member of the Board and at least two members (other than the charging or charged parties or any possible witnesses) from the local area involved. This Investigating Committee or representatives thereof shall make one or more local visits of investigation of the complaint. After full investigation following due process and offering the charged party(ies) opportunity to defend him or herself, the Committee shall report its findings and recommendations to the Board of Directors for action.

c. The charged party(ies) shall have free access to all charges and evidence cited against him or her, and shall have full freedom to defend him or herself before the Investigating Committee and the Board, including the right to legal counsel.

d. Recommendation made by the Committee shall be:

1. Advice that the charges be dropped as unfounded
2. Specified admonishment
3. Reprimand
4. Dismissal from membership

2. Should a member of this Association be expelled he or she shall at once surrender his or her membership certificate to the Board of Directors. Failure to do so shall result in such action as legal counsel may recommend.

3. Should a member of this Association be expelled from another recognized professional association or his/her state license revoked for unethical conduct, the Standing Committee on Ethics shall investigate the matter and, where appropriate, act in the manner provided above respecting charges of unethical conduct.

4. The Committee will also give due consideration to a formal complaint by a non-member.

SECTION V. PUBLIC INFORMATION AND ADVERTISING

All professional presentations to the public will be governed by the Standards on Public Information and Advertising.

I. TELEPHONE DIRECTORY LISTINGS

Yellow Pages. All listings should be governed by the principles of dignity, modesty and uniformity.

A. Special type (boldface, etc.) and lined boxes or any other technique tending to make one individual or firm's listing stand out from other listings in the directory is a breach of professional ethics.

B. A proper listing will include no more than the following:

(1) Name
(2) Highest earned relevant degree (one only)
(3) State licensure (including license No.)
(4) AAMFC clinical membership
    (Diplomate status if attained)
(5) Address
(6) Telephone number
(7) Designated specialty

C. Office hours (or the statement "By Appointment Only") may be listed if permitted by the local telephone company.

D. Any title including words such as "Institute," "Center," "Clinic," "Service" is acceptable only if a group practice includes at least three professionals. Other AAMFC members of such a group may choose to be listed under the identifying group practice name as well as separately in the proper alphabetical location.

E. When titles utilizing the name of a city, county, or state are employed, care should be taken to indicate the private nature of the enterprise.

Sample Individual Listing

Jones, John J.
    M.A.
    Member, American Association of Marriage and Family Counselors
    By Appointment Only
    123 N. Main 672-3903
    Res. 324 S. Adams. 674-2811

Sample Group Practice Listings

(a) Jones, John J. and Associates
      Patricia Adams, Ph.D.
      John J. Jones, M.A.
      Richard Williams, D. Min.
      123 N. Main 672-3903

(b) North Main Family Institute
      Patricia Adams, Ph.D.
      John J. Jones, M.A.
      Richard Williams, D. Min.
      123 N. Main 672-3903

(c) North Main Family Institute
      John J. Jones, M.A.
      123 N. Main 672-3903

(In this example Patricia Adams and Richard Williams will be listed alphabetically elsewhere with the same address and phone number as North Main Family Institute.)

II. PRINTED PROFESSIONAL MATERIALS

A. *Stationery, Business Cards and Announcements.* Dignity and good taste should characterize the printed professional materials of an AAMFC member. Select paper stock, type and composition suitable to the presentation of a professional practice. Imprinting should be limited to a minimum of simple, clearly legible information:

(1) *Name and degree.* Listing more than the highest earned relevant degree rarely adds information and detracts from the dignity. Listing an honorary degree (D.D., D.Sc. etc.) is a violationg of professional modesty. Using the title "Dr." in front of one's name, in place of or in addition to initials of a doctoral degree following the name, is considered improper.

(2) *Type of practice.* The AAMFC member will ordinarily identify himself/herself as a Marriage and Family Counselor. Related professional identification may be included (Licensed Clinical Social Worker, Licensed Psychologist, etc.)

(3) *Specialty.* Should a member wish to emphasize a single specialization within marriage and family practice, he or she may do so provided the designation reflects an exclusive emphasis.

(4) *AAMFC membership.* Persons holding clinical membership in the AAMFC may designate this by the following statement: "Member, American Association of Marriage and Family Counselors."

(5) *Address and telephone.* The location of the professional practice may be designated by appropriate address and telephone number(s).

(6) *Insignia.* Professional insignia intended to convey the orientation or focus of professional practice may be proper if the design and content is simple and informational.

B. *Brochures.* The production and distribution of public informational materials is an appropriate activity of the marriage and family counselor. The purpose of such material is to inform the public, not to "promote" the individual's practice. Therefore the emphasis should be on simple statements of services offered, factual presentations of the practitioner's relevant training and experience, and accurate information about contracts and conditions for service.

The Seed Principle:
The Secret Of A Dynamic Private Practice

Before leaving the subject of standards that govern your work, let me share with you what I believe to be the secret of success in any dynamic practice. This principle is not spelled out in the ethical guidelines just mentioned, but I believe that it is implied.

I learned the principle and applied it to our own practice after some careful thought about tomatoes. Yes, tomatoes! While harvesting bucket after bucket of sweet cherry tomatoes one season from our garden, I remembered that they all had sprung from one tiny seed. It occurred to me that because I did not selfishly hoard that seed for myself, but gave it up to the earth, because of that *giving* act, I now had more tomatoes, and seeds, than I could use. The principle of one seed turning into thousands struck me like light flooding a dark room. And it occurred to me that this same principle of nature and of God must also work in the realm of professional and interpersonal relationships.

So we began to apply the seed principle of giving freely of our services to those who could not afford $50 per hour as a kind of *in vivo* research experiment. We set aside certain hours each week for "free clinic"-type service and gave away our time and skill at little or no charge. In addition, we began to give those patients who could afford the fee extra time when needed during a particularly difficult session. Other programs of "going the extra mile" with our patients were also begun at that time.

The results? For a while (the germination stage) we saw no evidence of any tangible change in the practice, aside from our own personal joy in giving and the wonderful things that happened to our patients' lives. But it was not long before the rate of referrals to our practice began to grow dramatically and steadily. And these were patients who could well afford the full fee! All of the new referrals were not directly traceable to the "no-charge" work, but neither had we done any other practice promotion work during this time interval!

I have no statistical evidence to present to you to support the effectiveness of the seed principle in private practice. I can only share with you the outcome of three years' consistent application of this strategy. And without reservation I believe that over and above all the methods that we will outline in this handbook, the seed-giving principle does more to stimulate growth in any practice when it is applied diligently and liberally.

Whether you have an adequate practice now, or you are now preparing to enter that world, we strongly urge you to commit yourself to *giving away your services, your time, your energy, and your compassion* to those who are needy. Common sense would tell you to expend all your efforts seeking only those "paying patients." But as we know in our profession, common sense doesn't always produce results! The seed-giving principle is paradoxical — BUT IT WORKS!*

And note the guarantee that accompanies this ethical standard of conduct. It says this:

> *"GIVE, and it will be given to you:*
> *good measure, pressed down,*
> *shaken together, running over*
> *will be put into your lap.*
> *For the measure you GIVE*
> *will be the measure you get back."*

---

*For a more in-depth explanation of the series of events which led the author to this discovery, please refer to "A Personal Discovery", page 213.

CHAPTER FOUR

HOW TO GAIN RECOGNITION
IN YOUR COMMUNITY

CHAPTER 4
HOW TO GAIN RECOGNITION
IN YOUR COMMUNITY

We come now to that most important process of reaching out to your community to let them know about *you*. We hear much in the news these days about having a "low" or a "high" profile with the public. One's profile with the people simply means how well known he is in his community, and how hard he works at gaining that level of recognition. This concept is vital to developing a successful independent practice.

One of the most powerful means by which a mental health professional can increase or achieve a "high" profile in his community lies in presentation making. Whether you are just beginning your practice, or you have a well-established one now, you want to let as many groups and individuals in your area as ethically possible know about you, your skills and your availability to them. In this chapter we will consider how to prepare for and set up a presentation program to build your practice.

Preliminary Preparation To Presentation Making

Many of us become so caught up in professional jargonese from so many years in school and our own in-group circles of therapist friends that we forget how to talk everyday street talk. We need to take the time to shift gears and train ourselves to communicate in a clear, informal, and natural manner so that we can reach all levels of people, the educated and the uneducated, the rich and the poor, the professional and the layman.

Before we come to strategies for presentation making and how to set up the presentation, take some time here to examine these questions. After reading the question and considering your answer, jot down possible answers to each question as if they were actual responses that you were giving to a member of the audience at a presentation. These are questions that are asked over and over again during the course of presentation making and it is likely that you will face them sooner or later. Respond to each question in simple, direct, lay language, as if you were talking to the typical high school graduate. Just to be sure you are truly communicating, you might check out your answers to see if they are understood by a lay friend or someone in your family.

Here are the most commonly asked questions of the mental health professional:

What is therapy all about?

"What's the difference between a psychiatrist and a psychologist? A marriage counselor and a social worker?"

"Does counseling or therapy *really* help?"

"Who needs therapy, anyway?"

"How long does counseling take?" (Be prepared for this one; it is a favorite among potential and new patients alike).

"What kind of people go into therapy?" (Try here to define the patient in a positive, hopeful, "non-crazy", and non-clinical manner).

"What goes on in therapy?" (CAUTION: Use as little clinical jargon as possible).

"How do you know when you need therapy?"

"How do you go about finding a therapist?"

"Well, I have a friend who was in therapy for years, and it didn't help her one bit. How do you explain that?"

"What do you do if the wife is willing to come in and work on the marriage problems, but the husband will not?"

"We have a problem teenager who refuses to come for counseling. Would it do any good for just my husband and me to come in?"

What makes YOU special?

A key to getting referrals is letting people know what you do that is special TO THEM or a loved one. It is simply not enough to say, "I am a therapist with a private practice and I help people with emotional problems." That's much too general and does little to relate to a specific individual need. The following questions should help you pinpoint what it is that *you* do that dove-tails with human needs. And again, use the casual, down-to-earth style in responding.

(1) What specific problems, symptoms or behaviors do you work best with? Get the best results with?

(2) Do you prefer to work with males or females?

(3) What age groups do you enjoy working with most of all? Children? Adolescents? Young adults? Adults? The elderly?

(4) Do you work more comfortably with individuals? Couples? Families? Groups (How large? Type? Problem area?).

(5) When do you feel the *least* comfortable and with whom?

Males or females? What age group? How many patients seen together in a group? What specific symptomatology or disorder? What racial or ethnic group? (This question is not the most popular one to ask, but it is essential that we face up to it).

What Makes YOU Interesting?

Is there anything about you, your background, the problems you deal with, the people you see, or the opinions you hold — what about *you* would make a group of people want to listen to you talk to them for an hour or so while they sit on hard, uncomfortable folding chairs!? Perhaps the following questions will suggest to you some ways your work is a bit colorful and just a bit different from the therapist across the hall (who may speak to them next month!).

(1) Describe the most unusual case you have ever treated? (Keeping confidentiality in mind, describe the history, development, what problems it caused, how was it unusual, how was it common, what was the course and outcome of therapy, and associated anecdotes).

(2) What research have you done that would interest the layman?

(3) What innovative treatment methods or strategies have you developed that a layman would identify with?

(4) Do you hold any controversial position in your profession? (e.g., Alcoholics becoming social drinkers; heroin addicts being treated successfully; treating the spiritual and physical needs of the patient as well as the emotional; etc.).

(5) How would you treat some of the most common problems within the community? (e.g., overeating, smoking, depression, marital conflicts, sexual dysfunction, parent-child conflicts, reducing stress, and so on). Can you offer short-term training or treatment in any of these or others?

(6) What personal experiences in your own background, training, or practice would make for colorful anecdotes?

(7) What have you learned from your patients over the years?

(8) What life-changes have you made that have changed you as a person? That have given you the most happiness and peace? (NOTE: SELF-DISCLOSURE IN PRESENTATION MAKING IS A MUST!).

You are well armed for any presentation situation when you have taken time to deal with these issues and questions. Now, let's take a closer look at the matter of using the presentation approach to expand the practice.

Presentation Work — A Key To Referrals

Recently, a member of our family had a new home built. Upon moving in he discovered that there was no running water in the kitchen sink. He did not get on the phone and call the water company and complain about the lack of water in the reservoir or problems at the pumping station. What did he do? He simply assumed that there must be some problem in the pipelines that connected his sink to the water supply. He found that the plumbers had failed to connect the sink to the main line; he made the connection, and the problem was solved.

In building referrals and introducing yourself to your community you need to make the same assumption, and the same connection. You need to assume that the "reservoir" of potential patients is more than adequate to sustain your practice. You need to create a means by which you can tap into that reservoir in the community and provide a channel for them to flow into your practice. The presentation, like the pipeline, is a vital link.

Appearing before various groups in your area gives you the opportunity to accurately represent your profession to the public. The average layman's conception of the mental health professional is based on what he sees on comedy programs on TV, or the image he perceives from the "talk show psychologists." Neither example is likely to move the person to seek help, unfortunately. But the presentation gives you an important opportunity to tell them what the profession stands for, to demonstrate the dignity and ethical reliability of your work, and to help them see that their lives can be improved through mental health services. And all of this is accomplished in an entertaining, informal style centered around some major topic of interest.

Presentations also offer you the possibility of reaching out and serving a larger number of individuals at one time. You can share information and insights that give hope and direction to human lives. The objective of any presentation should always be *service.* The emphasis should be to provide professionally sound information in as detailed and concrete a manner as possible. You don't seek referrals in your presentation work. You seek to *serve* — the referrals come as a happy byproduct of your freely giving of your knowledge and time.

One final point before we move into some tips on presentation making: Remember: the presentation is a reciprocal process. You appear before the group and provide professional information and help at no charge. In turn, the group provides a channel by which you can communicate your personality, your skills, and your availability. They need you and you need them. You are serving one another and everyone profits from the evening's time together!

Tips On Making Effective Presentations

We have all spent enough time struggling to stay awake in the classroom, in workshops, or at conventions to know that not all public speakers are inspiring. But we also have witnessed those speakers who seem to have a way of keeping the audience in the palm of their hand throughout the meeting, and whose message rings in our ears long after the talk.

What's their secret? Exactly how do they do it?

Here are just a few of those things that should help you put "life" into your presentation to hold the interest of any group (and keep snoring at a bare minimum!).

(1) Be personal. As you address the group, make an effort to speak not to the group, but to each member *individually,* as if you were carrying on a one-to-one conversation. Use the phrase, "As you know . . . " often in your talk.

(2) Get eye contact. As you scan the group, try to get eye contact with as many people as possible.

(3) Weave self-disclosure throughout the talk. Let them know you as a human being. When appropriate, use your own life experiences as ways to illustrate your point. Don't be afraid to reveal your own limitations and weak points — it tends to make you more believable and "real."

(4) Use vivid anecdotes, analogies and stories. One good parable or story is worth a thousand abstractions! Anecdotes and analogies help to create mental pictures that captivate interest and hold an audience. It is a good idea to work up a repertoire of interesting stories to mix into your outline as your prepare for the talk. And add a bit of humor here and there — but don't overdo it.

(5) Be concrete. Keep abstract points to an absolute minimum. Give easy-to-understand examples from everyday life to illustrate

your material. In outlining your talk, try to include one good example (word picture) under each point.

(6) Don't read your presentation to the audience. Do you remember those profs who read their dusty lecture notes verbatim to you? How much did you learn? Use an outline if you must, but practice talking informally, extemporaneously and naturally.

(7) Use the audience as your barometer of success. Watch their faces and body language. If you note signs of confusion, restlessness, yawns, or disinterest, take it seriously. Pause, take a drink of water, give a concrete example to illustrate what you were saying, or pause and ask if there are any questions. This gets them participating and breaks the didactic monologue.

(8) Project enthusiasm! Smile! Talk with your arms and hands and body. If the sound system permits, move your location from place to place as opposed to standing stationary behind the podium. Enthusiasm is projected with the voice, face and body — it is contagious and convincing!

(9) Give out handouts. Prepare a handout that summarizes your major points and suggests practical methods to meet human needs. You can also print your name, address and office phone number on this handout for their future information.

(10) Talk their language. As noted earlier, keep the use of professional, psychological jargon to a bare minimum. Use simple language. You can judge by the number of yawns-per-minute how well you are communicating! Thoreau probably had this in mind when he said, "Simplify, simplify, and get closer to the truth."

(11) Utilize audio-visual aids. The use of movies, slides, videotape and audiotape add much to hold the interest of any group. A good rule of thumb is to lecture no more than 70% of your allotted time and use ancillary aids during the remaining time.

(12) Try to end the presentation with some form of group involvement. Some speakers use the question-and-answer period to end the talk. This tends to involve the more assertive members of the group, but misses the mark with the others. Giving the group a simple questionnaire similar to the type that you find in popular magazines always gets their interest. They are asked to mark "yes" or "no" responses on a quiz you design that helps them pinpoint their own needs in the area of your topic. Some speakers have used a period of guided imagery or role playing effectively in generating

active involvement and interest. Be creative in your planning to include the audience in your presentation — they love it!

How To Arrange Presentations

In order to appear before a group to present yourself and your topic you must first be invited to appear! How do you get invited?

There are three effective means by which you can become known in your area as an available speaker: (1) you can tell them yourself via an announcement of your area of specialization; (2) you can let a local speakers bureau know of your availability; or (3) you can employ a professional public relations person to tell them. Let's examine these methods in order.

The Presentation-Topic Announcement. As the title implies, here you merely prepare a brief and attractive brochure describing yourself and your topic. Your professional qualifications and specialization are outlined in brief. The topic or topics of interest to the community are then listed with short descriptive summaries of the message you can deliver. Information on how to contact you is then printed on the announcement and they are mailed to various groups in your community. An extensive cataloguing of target groups is provided for your use in Chapter 5.

A word of advice: When preparing your announcements, keep them *specific.* For example, an announcement for a topic entitled "Counseling With Parents" would doubtless fail to generate interest in your services. But the topic "Training Parents How To Talk Effectively With Their Teenagers" would probably keep you busy for many an evening. Be specific. Be practical.

The Speakers' Bureau. Most communities have several central speakers' bureaus as a clearing house of sorts for those with expertise in something. Colleges and universities typically maintain speakers' registers and are sometimes open to non-staff listings. Other possible sources for listing your services include hospitals, churches, libraries, and volunteer service bureaus. If you have difficulty locating the local speakers' bureau, simply call one of the local service groups (e.g., Lions, Masons, Rotary Club, etc.) and ask if they can help you locate this service. They may even be interested in your work themselves!

The Public Relations Professional. Some therapists are a bit uneasy about personally telling their community that they are available. Although the practice is completely ethical, some find it difficult to promote themselves.

And there are others who just do not have the time or know-how to do the leg work.

If you are among this group you may want to consider hiring a person who is trained to bring various segments of the community together. The public relations person has a wealth of experience and knowledge of the organizations and groups who could use your skills. He also knows many people in strategic positions in the community.

Where do you find a reputable PR person? You could go out and hire a local PR firm to represent you and arrange presentation engagements. But this is extremely expensive — and unnecessary.

An effective means to locate a PR person who is trained in working with professionals is through your local hospital. Call the community relations department in your nearby hospitals. Tell them about your practice, your topic(s), and your desire to set up a presentation schedule in the area. This is an excellent way to obtain highly skilled *and inexpensive* help in plugging into the main stream of the community.

It is vitally important to keep in mind that in addition to representing you, the PR person also indirectly represents your profession. Therefore, work closely with them and screen *everything* that they propose to present to the public on your behalf. If they are to make a verbal presentation of your work in introducing you to a particular group, ask them to first role-play a demonstration for you. It is essential that no mis-information or exaggeration of services be disseminated. The PR person is your agent and must be directed to uphold the highest degree of professional excellence.

Should you have no success in locating the right PR person through hospital channels, there is another source of low-cost help. Get in touch with the chairman of the marketing or business administration department at your local university. He can surely refer you to the best person. Most graduate students in public relations would jump at such an opportunity.

You are now well versed on the nuts and bolts of preparing to reach out to your community to serve them and build your practice. Let's move directly into the business of identifying target groups in your area that are good sources of referrals.

CHAPTER FIVE

GETTING REFERRALS FROM THE COMMUNITY

CHAPTER 5
GETTING REFERRALS FROM THE COMMUNITY

The other night my wife and I stopped by a local restaurant to celebrate a night out without the kids! The waiter brought the menu and left us to the work of decision making. The menu was a virtual catalogue of everything from A to Z in Mexican cuisine. To anyone who was in the least bit indecisive, this could certainly be the source of conflict.

So we narrowed down the field, made our selection, called the waiter, and ordered. A few minutes later our dinners arrived (and we are still dieting to this day!).

What does this have to do with getting referrals? Only this. You are about to explore many alternative selections that you must choose from in reaching out to your neighbors. Like the menu, you will not find every "dish" to your taste. Some will be too spicy. Some too expensive. Others too foreign or "weird." And still others will need to be put off till some later time. In any case, what follows in this and the chapters to follow are offered for your consideration as proven recipes for generating referrals.

You might first scan the items proposed. Check off those that seem most applicable in your area and those that you could comfortably implement. And then, reconsider the choices that you ruled out. Take some of the limits off of your imagination and try to project the idea into operation for yourself. Mentally rehearse putting the particular plan into action. You may be surprised to find that the "outrageous" scheme becomes the "outstanding" possibility.

As you read and ponder these methods and target groups, modifications and extensions of these ideas will occur to you that are particularly appropriate and sensitive to your community. When this happens please do not try to keep the idea in your head. If you do it may be lost forever. When you hit on some innovative twist to these suggestions, *immediately* jot it down in the margin or in the back of this manual. Then at some later time you will have the idea preserved for your attention and development.

Here then is the "menu" of those most effective and choice recipes that increase the flow of referrals to your practice* ... ENJOY!

---

*To help simplify and plan your contacts with these key sources of new referrals to your practice, refer to information on pp. 234-237.

Everyone A Potential Referral Source

It is unethical to directly solicit patients for our work. That is, we are forbidden to walk up to someone and identify them as a person with a problem and then to offer ourselves as the therapist. That's a professional NO-NO (See Chapter 3).

But when someone approaches you and asks what you do and requests your services this is, of course, a proper occasion to offer your help. If you have a positive, friendly and warm personality, and if you take a genuine interest in those you meet every day, then you will be asked the question, "What kind of work do you do?" on a regular basis. There are so few people today who take the time to really listen and sensitively care about another human being, that you will stand out like a cool breeze on a hot summer day!

Wherever you encounter people you encounter people with problems. You will be asked for your professional business card in the strangest ways and in the most unlikely places. We have been asked for our card at church, at parties, at baby showers, in the restroom, at the gas station, at the barber shop, and even once at a garage sale!

In addition to a smile and a lot of compassion in your daily relationships in your community, carry a good supply of business cards with you. You will need them.

Community Mental Health Organizations

Many communities have set up groups of laymen and professionals who meet together to improve the mental health services in their area. You might check into such groups and consider becoming actively involved. You have much professional insight to contribute. Others in your area who are concerned about quality care will also have an opportunity to meet you and learn of your work. Often such groups are formed around a particular problem that might interest you; for example, special interest groups in schizophrenia, the retarded, homeless children, alcoholism, drug addiction, the elderly, etc.

Free Clinics

The free clinic approach to providing medical and psychological services is becoming commonplace. Doubtless in your own community there are free clinics per se, emergency shelters, halfway houses, rescue missions, or no-cost treatment for alcoholics. In volunteering your services you have the opportunity of providing quality care to those who cannot afford it. You learn the art of working with minority groups.

As we noted in Chapter 3, in giving away your skill and time, you plant the seeds that yield a steady flow of referrals to your practice. Any time you spend in free clinic work will return to you multiplied many times over. Providing this type of work is typically what makes a practice flourish while others just "get by." It is in GIVING that we receive!

Telephone Hot Lines and Emergency Services

The hot line and the suicide prevention service have been established in nearly all major cities. Most use volunteer phone counselors who work out of their own homes, or answer phones at a central office. Excellent training programs are available to you at no charge. This is a fine means of offering your experience and training. You may consider becoming a phone counselor yourself. Or perhaps you could assist the local hot line in training volunteers.

Hot lines and suicide prevention services do a great deal of referral of callers to local therapists. Call your neighborhood hot line and ask if they would like to list you as a source of help for their callers. And remember: To build professional good will, *always* send the referring agency a letter of acknowledgement to indicate that the caller came for his or her appointment, and that you are grateful for their confidence.

In Chapter 8 we'll discuss the possibility of setting up your own hot line as an adjunct service to your practice.

Fraternal Organizations

Social and benevolent clubs are eager to have expert speakers address their members. The Masons, Eastern Star, Moose Lodges, Rotary, Lions, Knights of Columbus, and the Kiwanis Clubs are all good places to offer your services. You can approach such groups first as a member and later as an expert speaker, or simply come as an outside guest speaker. Once you appear before one such group you will likely be asked back again. Your name will also be passed along so that you will receive invitations from sister groups in outlying areas. So it is not necessary to call on a series of clubs under the same parent organization. If your topic is fresh and practical, they'll keep you busy!

Public Libraries

In case you haven't noticed, public libraries have changed. They are more than book depositories! They now offer paintings to borrow, records, tapes, audio-visual aids, and even present expert speakers on selected nights. When you have selected a few ultra-practical topics that would have widespread public interest or appeal, meet with the head librarian of your local library. Offer your services at no charge for an evening. You might also explore with him or her what topics they would recommend as possible areas for you to cover in a talk. The librarian has a finger on the pulse of society as he watches what the public is consuming in the way of reading material. Use this wisdom . . . it's free!

The Mass Media

Whenever you are scheduled to present a topic of public interest to any group, remember that your local newspaper editor may be interested. Prepare a brief announcement, "blurb" sheet describing in simple language your upcoming presentation. State how the talk will meet a given human need. If the meeting is open to the public, say so. Call your local newspaper and ask the name of the appropriate editor to whom you should submit this notice for public information (e.g., the health editor, the medical-science editor, etc.).

Have you noticed in recent years the number of psychologists, psychiatrists and marriage counselors who have entered the "Dear Abby" arena? In most popular magazines and newspapers you will find some form of self-help or advice column. If you have a flair for simply and candidly responding to "What do you do when . . . " questions, consider initiating your own column. Some professional people are now even conducting call-in talk shows on radio and TV here in Southern California. Is there a need for such services in your area?

Keep in mind when considering these suggestions that you may need help planning and breaking into this world. A good public relations person can help smooth out rough areas and open doors that we know nothing about (see Chapter 4, pages 62-63).

Using mass media is a powerful means by which to serve many thousands of people in an efficient manner. It also provides the vehicle by which to build a thriving practice. But as is the case in all our planning and outreach methods, we must keep things in perspective. We are first and foremost living and breathing representatives of our profession. When using the media, let the public see the highest level of professional conduct in all we say, write or do. We all have seen what happens when members of our profession become entertainers first and professionals last! If this suggestion holds your interest you might return to Chapter 3 and review the ethical standards as they pertain to the media.

The "Yellow Pages"

It has always amazed me that anyone would attempt to seek help with their most intimate emotional problems by randomly, hit or miss style selecting any therapist whose name sounds suitable. But experience has proven that some folk do just this! They turn to the Yellow Pages in their phone books and when they come to a name that sounds like the "right" ethnic group, race, sex, or sophistication, or, when the spot a degree of association membership that rings a familiar bell, they pick up the phone and say, "I'd like an appointment with. . ." knowing nothing more than that!"

Experience (ours and others) has shown, however, that the Yellow Pages do not produce a significant number of referrals compared to other methods of outreach, but it does bring in some. You could count on approximately 6% or less of overall referrals. But even if you should receive one patient per year via this method, the investment is still justified financially.

For example, in one local Southern California directory you can list your practice under one heading for an entire year for only $24. Over 300,000 homes receive this directory! Should one patient happen to like your name in the Yellow Pages, the first session alone pays the bill!

Here are some tips for listing your practice in the Yellow Pages. (1) Due to the minimal response, keep your listings to a minimum — one or perhaps two major headings. (2) List your name ONLY

*For a more in-depth course in practice Public Relations, Promotions, and Publicity, write to Duncliff's for more information.

under those headings under which you are duly licensed by the state to practice. (3) List your name, highest degree, address, and phone number. (4) If permissible, list your membership in professional organizations, such as APA, NASW, AAMFC, etc. (5) If you are a board diplomate list this under your name (although the average person will find no meaning in it). (6) Consider placing your name under alternate headings; for example, Clinics, Alcoholism Treatment & Education, Drug Treatment Centers, Marriage & Family Counselors). (7) NEVER use display or block advertising. (8) Consider placing your name in other directories in nearby areas. (9) Many State and local professional associations list their members under their own name: e.g., "Los Angeles County Psychological Association Members." Contact your local group and inquire into the cost of placing your name under their umbrella.

In summary I want to remind you to keep your advertising expense in this area as low as possible but still making your name visible under your major heading. And most importantly, before placing any ad, *review Chapter 3* and/or consult with your professional organization for more detailed guidelines.

Churches and the Clergy

In recent years there has been a virtual explosion of interest in church-sponsored marriage encounter and marriage enrichment retreats. The religious community now more than any time in history is accepting their responsibility to minister to the emotional needs of their flocks.

There are a variety of ways to approach the clergy. If you are an active member of a church, let your pastor or priest know that you have a private practice and what you specialize in. You might suggest to him that you run a group in the church centering around some area of human need. For example, you might propose a group on marriage enrichment, or how to bridge the generation gap, or a course in relaxation training, or how to apply the Bible to a marriage, or a program in behavioral weight control, or vocational planning, and so forth.

It is important in dealing with the clergy to let them know that you would be pleased to see those members of the congregation who cannot afford private therapy at a minimal or no fee. One therapist began his practice while working out of church office facilities at no charge to himself. In exchange, he agreed to see all patients for only a minimal charge and what the patient chose to contribute to the church itself. He now has a thriving practice and receives many full-fee patients through that church.

What about sending announcements of your practice to clergymen? This may result in some referrals, but don't count on it. Pastors are flooded with literature and your announcement will likely end up in the round file.

Clergymen are becoming increasingly aware of their *own* need to update counseling skills. Why not consider providing workshops for pastors in basic counseling skills? Topics which are in demand include series in crisis intervention, marriage counseling, working with the alcoholic and his family, ministering to the drug addict, courses in leadership psychology and decision making and so on. Consultation of this type provides an exciting dimension to your practice.

In Chapter 8 we will explore a spectrum of ideas and plans that can make a practice come alive!

Before leaving our discussion of the clergy let me point out something. The pastor or priest can become an important therapeutic ally in your work with the patient. If your patient reports that his problems have spiritual implications or in some way relate to his faith, consider calling in expert consultation. Regardless of your own spiritual persuasion, the pastor can function as a powerful co-therapist. Let him know that you are working with the patient (with the patient's consent) and ask if you might meet together so that you might put your heads together in helping him. You will facilitate the treatment process and add a potential source of new referrals to your practice as well.

Classroom Teachers

Teachers and students alike are often eager to have some new material injected into the classroom. Some sample topics which have proven successful include the following: Lectures and demonstrations on relaxation training before health education classes; biofeedback demonstrations with psychology classes; behavioral methods of weight control with nursing students, and the like.

Inform those teachers whom you know of your willingness to appear in their classes. You might also consider, if you are the bold sort, calling the department head or principal to offer your time and skills to his staff.

Parent-Teachers' Associations

Here's a likely group who would love to ask you some "tough" questions about how to live with kids! Let a friendly teacher or the school principal know of your availability.

Day Care and Preschool Facilities

There has been a boom in day care and preschool facilities of late. They encounter problem children (and problem parents!) every day. For a multitude of reasons, their staff is unequipped to respond to these needy people in a therapeutic way.

Have you considered offering monthly or biweekly discussion groups for parents and/or teachers? What about in-service training for the teachers on managing problem children? Put together an attractive and carefully planned brochure and send them out. Then follow up the mailing with a personal call to the director of the center. They may not be able to pay you a great deal, but those referrals that are a byproduct of your work there will make up for the lack.

Law Enforcement Agencies

Police, probation and parole, and protective agencies are showing an increased awareness of improving their own community relations skills. Some police departments now employ full-time psychologists.

What about proposing a program of in-service training for local law enforcement agencies? You might offer to run a series on crisis intervention techniques, or handling the drug addict, or even teaching the spouses of officers how to live this unique lifestyle. When you have outlined a potential program, get an appointment with the chief or director. It is always best to start at the top and work down!

Youth and Social Clubs

The YMCA, YWCA, Boyscouts, Girlscouts, Boys' and Girls' Clubs, Community Recreation Centers, and other such organizations often ask outside speakers to present practical know-how to their members. Some of the most popular topics for such groups include the following: Vocational planning, progressive relaxation training in overcoming negative habits, biofeedback training, communication training for marriage, premarital counseling, assertive training, child management workshops, self-hypnosis, and the list is endless.

Typically, a small fee is charged each member for your time. You will not get rich doing this type of work, but the referrals that follow will abundantly reward the investment of your skill!

Parents Without Partners

In Southern California, as in many other areas, the rate of divorce is as high as the rate of marriage; nearly a one to one ratio! Parents Without Partners (PWP) is a wonderful organization formed to meet the needs of the single parent. The many problems of the person who finds him or herself alone for the first time are innumerable. For example, problems of depression, loneliness, social isolation, social prejudice, child management crises, and others come to the attention of this group every day. PWP is most receptive to mental health professionals sharing their expertise with their members.

Either a phone contact from you or a carefully prepared announcement detailing your topic material should result in one or more invitations. Contact the president of the local chapter in your area. And when you outline topics that you are qualified to speak on, keep the needs of this special population in mind. The need for your help is desperate and immediate.

Retired Persons Associations

If you have knowledge and a big heart concerning the many difficulties confronting the elderly, here is a group that needs you. Problem areas include loneliness, grief and mourning of lost loved ones, managing pain, feelings of uselessness and hopelessness due to loss of work identity. Offer your services to local senior citizens or retired persons organizations — it is an enriching experience!

Foster Parent Programs

Operated through the social welfare departments, most foster care programs these days are devoting much effort to training foster parents in the art of child discipline and other areas of child care. Could you provide any training expertise on creative discipline methods? How to live with teens? Raising the retarded or handicapped youngster? Or perhaps teaching behavioral management techniques for the parent with the acting-out child?

Consider the needs of the foster children and parents. Then prepare a *specific* topic or topic series that you could present to foster parents. Present it to the agency director, or a service worker. Keep your fee as low as possible. The name of the game, again, is *SERVICE*. Referrals are automatic!

Child Abuse Programs

The child-abuser is now able to come out of hiding. Many groups are now openly providing services and a way to rechannel rage for these tormented parents.

Many of the workers in such groups are ex-abusers themselves. They have plenty of "firing line" experience, but little professional know-how. You might consider offering your skills in such areas as practical ways to handle impulse acting out, desensitization to reduce anxiety and fear, relaxation training, crisis intervention training for both workers and parents, or perhaps active listening techniques such as those taught in Parent Effectiveness Training. Or you might help these suffering people simply learn how to love and enjoy their children — and how to forgive themselves!

Back in the old days when people used to draw water from the well, a small amount of water was poured into the pump to start the flow. That is what I have attempted to do in this chapter. The ideas and target groups outlined here are meant not as the "last word" in possible points of outreach. They are designed simply to share with you a few of those "proven" methods, and are intended to prime the well of your creativity.

Before advancing to Chapter 6 where we explore professional referrals, pause here for a moment. Ask yourself these questions:

"Which of these groups are active in my community?"

"Which particular groups would be most likely to want my services in presentations or training seminars?" (List in ranking order).

"Who do I know now who may be able to help me get a foot in the door in these groups?"

"What topic(s) could I speak on with authority? With what groups are such topics most applicable?"

"This week I will contact _____ *to explore the possibility of speaking to that group."*

The last question carries an important message for you. That message can mean the difference between your success or failure in private practice. That message is a secret that you MUST LEARN if you ever intend to support your family by your own practice.

The message and the secret are contained in three small words. Here they are . . .

DO IT NOW!

After you have implemented at least one idea from this chapter, continue to the next chapter. And there too the secret to unlocking referrals from the professional community is the same. DO IT NOW!

DO IT NOW!

CHAPTER SIX

GETTING REFERRALS FROM OTHER PROFESSIONALS

CHAPTER 6
GETTING REFERRALS FROM OTHER PROFESSIONALS

We come now to the second major source of referrals that you should cultivate in building your practice. That is the professional community.

In reaching out to the community at large we emphasized that your first responsibility is that of *SERVICE*. The same holds true in introducing yourself to the professional sphere. You want to let other professional people know that you are skilled, qualified, and available to serve them and those they serve. In other words, you are not so much saying to the professional person, "I am in private practice and I need patients." You ARE saying, "If you have need of a trained and skilled mental health professional, I am ready to assist you in your work."

It may seem like hair splitting to stress this point. But I believe that many over-eager therapists lose countless referrals simply because they go at this process backwards. In their zeal to build a practice, they communicate to the professional person the message that centers on "I NEED." To establish a relationship that is conducive to the professional person making referrals, the therapist should always project the message, "HOW CAN I ASSIST YOU IN YOUR NEEDS?" *SERVICE is the engine. REFERRALS is the caboose!*

As we discuss together methods and approaches in dealing with your professional neighbors, keep this formula in mind. SERVICE first, REFERRALS follow. We are talking about a reciprocal relationship here. Or, as it is sometimes called, "You scratch my back, I'll scratch yours." If you successfully demonstrate your willingness to *serve* their needs, referring patients to your practice will become a natural consequence of your relationship. Service elicits referrals from professionals faster than any slick, Madison-Avenue promotional scheme could ever accomplish.

With that in mind, let's look at the most effective and efficient approaches. And remember: If while you are scanning these ideas a modification or extension of the suggestion should occur to you, WRITE IT DOWN IMMEDIATELY.

Make The Rounds!

Once you have located your office and have hung out your shingle (see Chapter 2), drop in and shake hands with all the professionals in your office building. In the most friendly way, tell them that you have moved in or are subletting with Dr. So-And-So and wanted to get acquainted since you are now "neighbors."

He will likely ask you what you do and what type of people you see. You can toot your own horn here a bit and summarize your work. But keep HIS work in mind. For example, if you are visiting a pediatrician three doors down the hall, you might talk about a particularly interesting case involving children. If you are saying "hello" to an attorney on the second floor, you might tell him about some of your work with alcoholics in diversion work, or any work you have done in child custody cases, etc. Or the gynecologist across the hall would surely be interested in your work in marital counseling and sexual dysfunction therapy.

Have plenty of business cards handy with you on making the rounds. You might wish to set up luncheon engagements with those with whom you sense a certain rapport. Taking the professional to lunch always builds good will . . . and it's tax deductible!

Sending Out Announcements

Common sense would indicate that sending out announcements of a new practice is a good idea. But as is the case in many real life situations, common sense is not always reliable.

It has been our experience and many other therapists have confirmed this, that the policy of mailing formal "open house" announcements to professionals is generally a waste of time and money. Unless the person knows you personally and respects your work, the announcement will likely end up lining someone's trash can before the day is out. For the newcomer to private practice then, we would recommend against this practice. You will find other methods to be discussed in this chapter more powerful and much less expensive!

If, however, you already have an established practice and you change your office location, then sending a "WE'VE MOVED" announcement is a must. It also may bring your name to their mind and/or a particular person whom they might refer to you. An "open house" to celebrate your new location may be a good idea. But we recommend that you send a minimal number inasmuch as the announcement is a poor instrument either of service or referrals.

Physicians

Whatever you do, don't rely on referrals from physicians to feed the family or pay the rent! You may receive an occasional referral, but they will doubtless be few and far between.

In short, physicians have been found one of the poorest sources of regular referrals to a private psychotherapy practice. However, there are some ways to reach them and increase the flow of patients. Let's look at a few.

Make it a policy in your practice to get the name and address of all your patients' personal physicians. Do this at the time of the initial intake examination. Ask the patient if he or she would permit you to discuss progress with their physician, if appropriate, and then get a signed release of confidential information from the patient (see Figure 1). Most patients are delighted to have their doctor involved in their therapy.

From time to time send the physician a summary of patient's progress in therapy, along with a copy of the release form. In your summary letter, indicate that you would be pleased to consult with him at any time should he have any questions or desire your assistance with patient's care. Should the occasion of medical attention come up, such as the need for medication review or for physical examination, you might call the physician personally to discuss it.

CAUTION: Keep in mind that most physicians are overworked and time is hard to come by. So keep all correspondence brief, succinct, and professional. Include diagnoses, major complaints, goals for treatment, progress summary and prognosis. If the patient has any identifying number with the physician, use it in your references to patient in the letter. If not, use date of birth.

These methods represent to the physician an unique service to his work with the patient. When he next sees a person who is in need of counseling, your name is fresh in his mind.

FIGURE 1. **AUTHORIZATION FOR RELEASE
OF CONFIDENTIAL INFORMATION**

(LETTERHEAD)

AUTHORIZATION FOR RELEASE
OF CONFIDENTIAL INFORMATION

RE:_____ Date of Birth:_____

This is to authorize _____

_____
(address)

to disclose and release any information, including psychiatric and psychological records, of the above-captioned individual to Dr. Charles H. Browning, who is authorized to discuss all matters pertinent to the progress of the patient.

This information is considered instrumental to the ongoing evaluation and treatment of this patient.

Data particularly requested include:

____ psychiatric information   ____ social welfare data

____ psychological testing   ____ rehabilitation records

____ educational records   ____ legal information

____ medical information   ____ other _____.

Date _____ Signature _____
                                                    (patient, parent, legal guardian)

_____
(relationship to patient)

_____
(witness)

Another effective approach is making a direct referral to the physician. It works like this. Many times you will encounter a patient who has no personal physician. The patient indicates an interest in finding a "good" doctor and needs immediate attention. You simply refer the patient directly to a local physician in whom you have confidence. You participate in the referral by calling the doctor personally and *briefly* summarizing the need, that you are treating the patient in therapy, and ask him if he can see them. If the phone call bothers you, consider dropping the physician a summary statement of referral with your diagnosis, goals for treatment, and a statement of your availability to him, if needed.

This is a fine way to initiate a *quid-pro-quo*, reciprocal relationship with a local M.D.

One group of child psychologists asked a local pediatrician if he would let them place their announcement of services in his waiting room. He agreed. The announcement was in the form of a questionnaire. The parents in the waiting room were asked to check off any of the topics listed that they would be interested in learning more about. For example, how to handle bedwetting, thumbsucking, pants-messing, aggression, speech problems, learning problems, discipline problems, and the like. The patients were then asked to print their names and address and phone number and indicate the time they could attend a seminar dealing with the subjects. A $10 charge was indicated for a series of 4 one-half hour group sessions.

This approach was to the physician's liking since it took much of the burden of such problems off of his shoulders. Does the idea appeal to you?

Other Therapists

Ideally, those of us who are well established in our own practices should look back and recall the "lean years." In doing so we should empathize with the newcomers and refer patients to their practices to help them over the hard times. Unfortunately this is the ideal and we live in a world of stark realities.

If you are a "seasoned" veteran in the world of private practice, why not begin referring patients to those who are just starting out? Someday they may return the favor to you!

If you are a newcomer, don't rely on the old-timers to fill up your appointment book. But there are ways of influencing them so that there is more probability of them doing so. Let's look at a few now.

(1) *Join professional organizations.* Attend meetings, workshops and conventions of local professional groups. Get to know those in private practice, especially those who have "well-nourished" practices.

(2) *Take a colleague to lunch.* Private practice gets lonely for some. Arrange to have lunch periodically or regularly with a more experienced therapist and use the time for supervision and to let him get to know you and trust your work.

(3) *Get your work in print.* Tell your professional colleagues what you do in a journal! We often develop effective therapeutic techniques or strategies but because of our laziness when it comes to research and writing, we never seem to get them published. And I am the president of that club! But we must take the time and make the time to share what we have discovered with the professional community. This is our responsibility professionally. Once you have managed to get through the rewrites and the rewrites of the rewrites, you can then present your findings locally. Present your paper at a local or national convention. In this way you will be meeting your responsibility to the field, and at the same time your reputation will become established. Referrals are a natural outgrowth of publishing and presenting!

(4) *Refer out.* You will be asked to help those who must be referred to someone else since their need is outside your area of competence. Never say, "I don't do that type of work," or "you'll have to find someone who specializes in . . . " GET ACTIVELY INVOLVED IN EVERY REFERRAL. Never allow a person to hang up the phone or leave your office without your assisting them in finding the best possible help. Should a caller or a patient need the services of a speech therapist, a reading instructor, a dentist, an attorney, a birth control clinic, or even another therapist, take it upon yourself to assist in the referral. If you know of no one, research it for the person. Find out who is most respected and competent, call or write the professional person and pave the way for the referral. And after the referral is made, follow it up with a short summary of the referral information *in writing.*

This may seem like much unnecessary work on your part, but remember: Because you gave freely of your time and effort and concern you will somewhere down the line reap from what you have sown. The process of referring out typically results in reciprocal referrals. Every act of giving will return to you multiplied — often in new referrals to your practice!

(5) *Become an internship facility.* Offer your practice and your services to the local university counseling programs for a possible internship or practicum placement setting. Most program heads are always looking for good practicum placements.* And if your office is near the school where you did your graduate work, don't forget to let them know of your work and availability.

---

*Check with your state licensing board for any "red tape" relating to intern or assistant certification.

Hospital Staff Membership

Have you considered becoming a staff member of a local hospital? As a mental health professional staff person certain benefits are open to you. Should you have the occasion to admit a patient to the hospital, your staff status greatly facilitates your patient's care. In addition, you are exposed to many other professionals and you become more "visible" as a referral source for outside therapy. Don't overlook the opportunities open to you in terms of presenting training programs in your specialty in the hospital. Again, the exposure will show itself in your practice growth.

Health And Welfare Service Agencies

Many public health and welfare agencies use outside sources to complement their own services. They refer to independent practitioners for ongoing psychotherapy, psychological testing and evaluation, intensive treatment of behavioral disorders, and consultation.

Those agencies who commonly use private therapists include the following: State Department of Rehabilitation; local Social Service or Welfare Department; Child Protective Services; Department of Adoptions and Foster Care; the Department of Probation and Parole; organizations concerned with the disabled (e.g., mentally retarded, cerebral palsy, etc.).

In the course of your work with any patient, should you learn that they are associated with any of these agencies, use this as a two-edged opportunity. Get the patient's signed consent and call the service worker assigned to your patient. Enlist them in your work with the patient as someone who knows the special needs of the patient and can provide you with expert information. Secondly, in reaching out to those people and agencies that serve the patient, you broaden the base of potential referral sources to your practice. We will devote an entire chapter to the subject of developing referral sources from your existing patient caseload (see Chapter 7).

Alcoholism And Drug Diversion Programs

During the past few years there has been tremendous interest in alcoholism and drug diversion programs in the legal system. In these programs the abuser-offender is offered a choice of alternatives to satisfy the penalty of his maladaptive behavior. He can spend time in jail and/or lose his drivers license. Or, he can opt to spend a year or more in a diversion program. It's obvious why the diversion option is so popular! Basically the diversion programs consist of counseling, education, and rehabilitation lectures.

Attorneys, judges, and law enforcement personnel are typically referring offenders directly to public agencies that offer the programs, and even to some private practitioners who have set up their own programs. You might consider setting up such a program (see Chapter 8). Or perhaps you can offer your services to existing programs as a consultant, providing testing and evaluation, therapy after termination of program, or training for the program staff.

Attorneys

If you find physicians to be poor referral sources, wait until you see the results from attorneys! The only reason this group is included here is because there is one area in which they sometimes show promise. As we noted above, the interest in the diversion alternative is mounting. Attorneys are looking for professional mental health persons who can assist them and their clients in planning for diversion help before the court appearance. You might consider, should you be interested in this form of service, preparing a brochure outlining your program and sending it to local attorneys. But let me again caution you. Do not spend much time or money or hope in this direction — an unreliable referral source at best!

Marital Conciliation Courts

Some states now offer marriage counseling as a part of the divorce court system. The hope is that the divorce itself might be avoided through such counseling. Typically the court counselor sees the couple for a designated number of sessions (usually five) and then refers the couple to a private or agency therapist to continue with them. Such court counselors have a referral panel list from which they select counselors for the couple to call.

Investigate having your name and practice listed with your local conciliation court.

Your Present Job

Don't overlook your present employment setting as a base from which to generate referrals. You will meet administrators, faculty, colleagues and students who will ask you from time to time about your own private work. *Without soliciting patients,* let them know that you are in private practice and have time available. If you work in an university setting, don't forget to let the staff of the counseling center know of your outside work. Your practice may provide open hours at times when the university counseling center is closed. This would fulfill an important need for the students.

Does your employer typically send staff representatives to community service groups, planning councils, and inter-agency staff meetings? Many do. Perhaps you could represent your employer at local mental health committees, alcoholism councils, church-related groups, speech and hearing groups, service groups, etc. Offering your services to your employer in these "extra-curricular" duties carries with it a multitude of "extra-curricular" benefits!

Employee Assistance Health Programs

Modern industry is becoming more concerned with the overall health care of its workers, in addition to their productivity. They have learned that the two are inseparable.

When you see a patient who is covered by an employee assistance or health program, consider the following approach as a matter of routine policy in your practice. Get in touch with the director of the program. Inform him that you are seeing someone from his company in treatment. Ask him (or his secretary) to help you serve the patient by: (a) sending you a copy of their program benefit plan for mental health services; (b) sending you a supply, if they will, of insurance forms to expedite service to patient.

If you approach this relationship in a professional, friendly, and cooperative manner your name will likely be the first to come to mind when an employee requests mental health services.

Many employee assistance program directors appreciate follow-up reports from the therapist after referring patients to them. Make it a policy to send such feedback, but be certain to get the patient's signed release (see Figure 1, p. 84) before doing so. It is a good idea to send periodic and regular reports updating the program director on patient's progress and prognosis in terms of work performance and/or readiness to return to work. You might set aside a specific time each month to prepare such short summary reports for the company — the time investment will pay rich dividends! Going the extra mile in providing information over and above your therapeutic services makes you stand out as someone who is unique in professional circles. Your appointment book will reflect the courtesy and special care you give away free!

By the way. Don't forget to take the employee assistance director, and his secretary, out to lunch from time to time. There's nothing like the personal (but professional!) touch to keep good will and a good referral flow nourishing a growing practice.

Let this collection of potential target groups and methods stimulate your creativity and imagination. Try to double the list by considering those persons and agencies in your own community and noting them in the back of this manual.

As you expand the list, ask yourself the question: "Have I done EVERYTHING professionally feasible to bring my services and my practice to the attention of this person (group, agency, etc.)?" And as you ponder the answer, get out your calendar for next week and schedule AT LEAST ONE approach from this chapter or from your own list as part of your "must do" list. DO IT NOW!

Having done this, let's move on to an exciting approach to building a successful practice. I call it the "Pyramiding Effect."

CHAPTER SEVEN

THE PYRAMIDING EFFECT
"Patients Generate Patients"

CHAPTER 7
THE PYRAMIDING EFFECT
"Patients Generate Patients"

The growth of a successful professional practice is much like getting up in the morning. At first it's a struggle. Just getting those feet on the floor is a major accomplishment. Then, after the shower, breakfast, drive to the office and innumerable cups of strong coffee, the day just seems to pick up and flow. You seem to build a momentum that carries you along.

There is a principle of *momentum* operative in the development of a private practice. During the initial stages things go a bit slowly. The would-be private therapist must spend much time in practice promotion (see Chapters 4 through 6) and his patience and confidence are sorely tested. But then he gets his feet on the floor, so to speak. The "roller coaster effect" begins to level out (see pp. 15-17) and he notices that the number of patients begins to stabilize and gradually increase. What a thrill it is when you reach this turning point in your own practice!

Although there is always some need for community and professional outreach on your part, when you reach the point that your work has a self-sustaining momentum, you can relax a bit. Your patients seem to generate patients!

In this chapter we will exmaine how this happens. What phenomena cause one patient to yield three? And three twelve, and so on. Let's also carefully consider how you can profit from a knowledge of this phenomenon, which I call the PYRAMIDING EFFECT.

The Pyramiding Effect

Simply defined, the PYRAMIDING EFFECT or principle assumes that each individual patient is a potential source of other patients to a professional practice. Every person coming for help brings with him or her a set of interpersonal relationships and associations. As a result of the changes that accrue in the patient's life, it is probable that selected members of this set of associations will become aware of the therapist's work. This awareness may then result in a request for therapist's service.

Patients entering a practice in such a way seem to demonstrate a multiple chain reaction. That is, one patient refers two close friends or relatives. Each of them, in turn, refer three or four of their loved ones to the therapist. And these individuals may account for their own referrals. So, from a single patient the therapist may find himself serving ten! Thus the name "pyramiding effect."

The essential thing for you to keep in mind is this. EVERY patient that you see represents a potential pool of individuals who need your help. This principle should be in the back of your mind during every intake, during the course of therapy with each patient, and during regularly scheduled practice review sessions (see Chapter 10).

And like any principle, to have any value it must be ACTED UPON. Let's consider together methods by which you can ACT ON the pyramiding effect . . .

Changed Lives Speak For Themselves!

Everyone today is desperately seeking peace of mind in a not-so-peaceful world. Whenever people see that a person has found a "better way" to manage his life, a happier and a more meaningful way of life, they are intensely curious. Perhaps they knew the "changed" person as he used to be — withdrawn, depressed most of the time, or a slave to some life-long habit pattern. Now they see a transformed and radiant life before their eyes. It's somewhat like an ugly worm crawling up a branch, wrapping itself up in a blanket shutting out the world for a while, and emerging as a beautiful butterfly! Others still crawling with their face in the dust look up and ask themselves, "How did he do it?" "I wonder if I could also learn to fly?"

If a therapist is touching human lives in such a way that his patients learn to "fly" and give up crawling, his patient flow will show it. And after all, aren't we in the business of teaching suffering humanity that they do not have to crawl any longer? That's what mental health is all about. Teaching people to "fly."

When marriages are healed and the divorce lawyer is dismissed; when parents and teenagers are talking and laughing again together; when alcohol is no longer a major part of the family's budget — when others see these transformations in your patients, they'll want to know who helped bring about the metamorphosis!

Changed lives speak for themselves!

In our own experience in private practice the "word of mouth" (or the word of a changed life) has proved to be the most powerful stimulus to new patients. Our own patients' "new" lives, changed attitudes, adaptive behavior patterns, and inner peace* account for the major proportion of new patients entering our appointment book. This finding is confirmed by other therapists, and by physicians and attorneys in private practice as well.

The therapist who is professionally competent, who has successfully worked through his own personal problems, and who genuinely and compassionately cares for his patients and treats them with dignity and respect, that is the therapist who will see the pyramiding effect at work in his practice. If any one of the above conditions is lacking or has been neglected, the pyramiding principle is short-circuited.

The "word-of-mouth" flow of patients into your practice is a highly sensitive and extremely accurate measure of the degree to which you have mastered the above factors. Professional competence and skillfulness in therapeutic techniques, personal stability, and a loving concern for your patients are all mirrored directly in those persons who come to you because of what they have seen about your work in your patients' lives!

How many times has someone recommended their physician to you with the words, "He's the best . . . a great doctor!" What makes them say this in recommending him to you? It's simply because (1) he is competent professionally and gets results, (2) he is positive and friendly, and (3) he goes the extra mile and demonstrates his concern for the patient.

In addition to contributing the most dramatically to the growth of the practice, patients that generate patients represent the greatest satisfaction to the therapist. There is no greater confirmation of a successful therapeutic relationship than to hear these words: "I would like to make an appointment with you, because of how much I've seen So-and-so change!"

---

*Please see Chapter 12, "A Personal Discovery" for a description of the author's personal search for inner peace, and the outcome of that search.

The Therapeutic Acknowledgement Letter

Whenever a former or current patient refers a friend or loved one to you, acknolwedge his or her trust and confidence in you, and in the process communicate to the patient in a therapeutic manner.

Send the referring patient a letter of gratitude. In this letter you express your appreciation for the referral and the confidence the patient has in your work. The patient is then told that the fact that this person has come in for help has other very important implications. First of all, the patient should know that others are *noticing* his or her changes and improvement. Secondly, that the patient's changes are positively *influencing* others and giving new *hope* to those who are suffering. And finally, because of the positive changes in the patient's life, others are able to *share* their need for help with them. This letter has a powerful therapeutic effect, as you can imagine.

A sample Therapeutic Acknowledgement Letter is presented in Figure 2 as a model for your consideration.

FIGURE 2. THERAPEUTIC ACKNOWLEDGEMENT LETTER

(LETTERHEAD)

17 July 1981

Dear _____:

This is just a note to express to you my sincere personal greetings, and an opportunity for me to say, "Thank You!"

I am really grateful for your trust and confidence in our work and for your referral of Mrs. _____ to me.

It is important that you know what part you played in helping her to seek help. As you already know, it's not an easy matter making that decision to enter therapy. But because of the positive changes that she has seen first-hand in *you*, she found new hope and encouragement. Whenever others see favorable changes in someone they begin to believe that their own lives can improve too.

It's an exciting thing to know that the progress that you have made has already had such a far reaching impact on others.

So, let me again say, THANK YOU, and WELL DONE! And give my best regards to your family.

With warmest regards,

Direct Intervention With Significant Others

It is common practice in many therapeutic orientations to bring the patient's significant others into the diagnostic or treatment process. The patient's spouse, children, parents, grandparents, relatives, friends, co-workers and supervisors see the patient in his everyday milieu. Invaluable information can be obtained from this "inner circle" of the patient's life.

Typically the patient is asked if he or she would like the therapist to see those persons who can contribute important data to the treatment relationship. If so, the patient makes the arrangements for them to call the therapist for the appointment. Significant others can be seen with the patient or separately.

In addition to gathering representative feedback for therapy, the therapist demonstrates his concern and competence to those involved with the patient's life. It has been our experience that most patients are eager to bring about this arrangement, and most of his loved ones are similarly cooperative. In our practice, the significant others are seen during one of patient's regularly scheduled sessions. They are seen separately and the primary patient commonly assumes responsibility for the fee.

Indirect Intervention With Significant Others

It is not always possible, for many reasons, to get those close to the patient to come into the office. Many people don't want to be seen anywhere near, much less coming out of, a "shrink's" office. For others being in the presence of a therapist is in and of itself threatening. Guilt over their role in the patient's problems can also keep them away. And problems in scheduling account for others for whom direct intervention is not possible.

In such instances two methods have been found to be most effective. The first is the Diagnostic Questionnaire. The patient is asked to help in the diagnostic process by asking a key person in his or her life to complete a questionnaire. The questionnaire is brief, simple, and is tailored to the respondent's relationship with the patient. The therapist can establish a working relationship with many important people in the patient's life without ever seeing them face to face.

A sample Diagnostic Questionnaire is presented here for your examination. This particular form was used with a husband who refused to participate in his wife's therapy. Although he would not come into the office, he did participate through the mail and the treatment process was greatly enhanced. Note carefully the brief introduction at the outset of the questionnaire. This is important as it motivates and assures the respondent, and demonstrates the genuine interest and concern of the therapist for his point of view.

FIGURE 3. DIAGNOSTIC QUESTIONNAIRE

Dear Dennis:

You can be of great help in my work with Marianne. It's important that I get the complete picture, to get your viewpoint, in order for me to understand and to help bring about rapid and lasting change. I really do appreciate your feedback and your ideas.

Would you kindly give me your reactions to the following "nosy" questions? I will use what you say in my work with her, toward the goal of re-establishing harmony in your life together.

1. Would you please give me *three* areas in which you feel Marianne could change which would make your relationship more happy? What specifically could she DO to make things better?

2. Applying the same question to you. What specifically do you feel that Marianne would like for you to DO to make your life together more happy and loving? (If you're stumped for an answer, just take a few "wild guesses").

3. Could you please tell me just how your relationship is different today as compared to the time just before and immediately after you and Marianne were married? What's changed? What's missing? What's better? (please be specific).

4. Sometimes bringing the family members together in a shared activity results in important changes. Are there any activities that you enjoy that you could include the children in with you? Are there any that you could teach them?

5. And likewise, what things do the kids do or get a kick out of that you might do *with them*? What could you learn from them? (I am always amazed how much I learn myself from my own little children!). In answering this one, try to see it from their standpoint: what makes them proud? What do they do well? What are their favorite games? And so on . . .

6. What unusual, different, "wild", or just plain crazy-sounding things have you thought about doing but you have never really made time for? Things that you feel would be fun or exciting, either alone or with Marianne. Which ones of these would you like to try with Marianne in the near future?

7. And finally Dennis, in my work with Marianne, what things do you think that I should know that might help me understand the situation? What would you like to see come of our work together? (PLEASE be open and frank. Speak your mind candidly, and feel free to make any suggestions or comments).

A second approach in reaching others important to the patient is via the telephone. Many times those who cannot or will not come into the office will agree to a telephone consultation. Typically the patient is instructed to set up the telephone interview in which the significant other calls the therapist at a specified time set aside for them. The patient assumes fee responsibility (regular session or half-session fee is charged). This method is sometimes preferred by those who fear putting their thoughts in writing. It also facilitates the development of rapport and a working relationship.

A combination of the questionnaire and the telephone interview may be possible. The therapist might first talk with the respondent and ask his cooperation personally. The questionnaire may then be sent out after a relationship has been initiated. Or perhaps the questionnaire might open a channel to call the respondent and discuss his answers — with the patient's consent, of course.

In addition to profound clinical data obtained through these means, you will be surprised at the results in terms of future referrals to your work. In offering to spend extra time on your patient's behalf, you increase the rate of progress, and at the same time, the rate of growth of the pyramid.

Pyramiding Potential

We have discussed elsewhere (see Chapters 5 and 6) the multiple avenues open to you in community and professional circles. Each patient whom you see in therapy brings with him or her a group of people, agencies, organizations, clubs, doctors, churches, schools, and so forth. Each person or group sees the patient as he functions in the real world. Each can provide you with important diagnostic data.

And as you collect this data on the patient's behalf and with his consent, keep in mind the pyramid potential of each contact. As part of your intake procedure, consider possible sources of outreach for your practice. During review of your caseload (see Chapter 10, pp. 153-156) ask yourself the question: "Who are those key persons who know the patient who could contribute information that might assist in diagnosis and treatment? — family, friends, co-workers, professional people, social and recreational influences, religious influences, educational involvements, etc. Actively involving key resources in the treatment process communicates much about you and the way you work. How many therapists do any more than simply see the patient once a week in the office, and no more? That's all most of us do and the public knows it!

What happens when a therapist gets involved in bringing many important others together to help the patient? Those important others see the extra care demonstrated and they do not forget it easily. When they find themselves, or a loved one, in need of help in a personal way, who do you think they will call? You're right. You.

The pyramiding effect begins with you. It rests on an attitude of *service.* But not "just enough" service to satisfy the fee. Patients generate patients in direct proportion to the degree to which you give more than you are paid to give. It sounds simplistic perhaps. And it is simple. Giving more than expected, although absurd to many, always results in multiplied returns! All you have to do to prove this in your own practice is to perform an experiment.

Give twice (or more) the service that you are expected to render for each session paid for. Make no charge or mention of your extra time invested for the patient, and then watch the results!

In essence, the secret of the effectual working of the pyramiding effect in your practice is threefold: (1) Maintaining a loving and compassionate concern for your patient; (2) Expressing that concern through an involvement of many significant others in the patient's therapy; and (3) Freely and generously giving of your time and energy on the patient's behalf.

This is how pyramids are built.*

We have now considered the three primary sources for practice growth, i.e., community, professional, and patient referrals. In the next chapter let's discuss the technology for maximizing the financial potential of an independent practice. A private practice can involve so much more than simply seeing patients in individual or group consultation. Let's look at some fascinating possibilities together — many of which you probably have never considered before . . .

---

* A Step-by-Step system for Pyramiding is found in Duncliff's *"How To Build A Practice Clientele Using Key Referral Sources—A Sourcebook."* See pp. 234-237.

CHAPTER EIGHT

METHODS FOR ACHIEVING
MAXIMUM INCOME POTENTIAL

CHAPTER 8
METHODS FOR ACHIEVING
MAXIMUM INCOME POTENTIAL

What do you think of when you think of a private practice? Most of us conceive of a therapist with his own office who sees patients either individually or in groups. He charges a set fee and all his time is spent in patient consultation. We assume that the therapist's income is produced entirely from patient fees. This image of the independent therapist is correct. But it only taps the surface of the potential of a successful practice.

It's like a tree. We can look at the tree and recognize its value as a thing that provides shade. Or we might climb it. We might see the possibility of building a tree house in its branches. But beyond that we typically see little value for that tree. We limit its potential by our own short-sightedness. That same shade tree that we labeled as only good for three things, has an infinite number of uses and benefits. It produced the desk that I am sitting at right now. It gave the material for my chair. The paper that you are holding in your hand came from that tree. And the pencil that you use to mark special points of interest in this manual, it was originally part of that tree. And so on. So then, a tree is more than a tree!

A private practice is more than a place to see patients!

In this chapter we will ask you to take off some of the preconceived notions that you might hold regarding what exactly one can do in his own practice. Open your mind to entertain new ideas about the sources of income possible through your own practice. Someone with vision and imagination had to look at the tree and see my desk, the paper, the pencil. Set your own creative imagination to "see" your own practice as a fertile milieu with endless potential for service and for generating income for your family.

Because most clinicians spend so much time preparing themselves professionally in the university, and then find themselves in direct clinical work thereafter, it is sometimes difficult to perceive opportunities in private practice other than clinical activities. Those therapists who have learned the multi-dimensional scope of a private practice typically have learned this over a long period of trial and error. And many of the opportunities and alternatives open to them were discovered by stumbling over them by accident.

This manual is designed to short-cut the trial and error, groping in the dark process for you. In this chapter I have brought together a spectrum of ideas, plans, methods and procedures which I have liberally borrowed from a pool of successful private practices. Inasmuch as it is impossible to trace the person of origin for each idea, no credit is given here. But on behalf of all of those who such methods profit, let me say a sincere THANK YOU!

Before we explore these methods in detail, let me again bring a vital principle to your attention. As clinicians we have a tendency to think theoretically, to ponder and to analyze information. In short, we tend to be more "head" oriented and less "action" oriented. But if we are to establish a growing practice, and if you are to get your money's worth out of this manual, you will have to resist this tendency!

The secret or effectivenss of any and all of the following procedures depends not in their cleverness or uniqueness. The secret for their usefulness rests on ACTION.

Please let me encourage you as strongly as I know how. As you read through this chapter, make yourself, force yourself, put yourself on a contingency contract if you must, but do whatever you have to do to put what you read into ACTION! A cookbook is a useless thing unless someone gets down to the business of acting on the recipe. As you read, DO IT NOW! DO IT NOW! If a particular idea strikes you as something that you believe you can apply, stop, get out some paper and pen, and plan how you can implement it. Do some brainstorming. Talk to colleagues about the notion. Or implement it on the spot.

If you are aiming high and desire the *reality* of a successful practice of your own, DO IT NOW! If you are interested in the *fantasy* of a practice of your own, just read through and then file this book with all the others on your book shelf. I think I've made the point; enough said.

Let's now examine those approaches which can dramatically increase the income in a private practice. If carefully applied, any one of the approaches in this chapter could support the practice, over and above patient fees. Not all the methods will suit your taste, of course. But when you find yourself saying to yourself, "That's a

great idea . . . I wonder if that would work in my practice?" Begin
IMMEDIATELY to explore its possibilities. And as you did earlier,
don't hesitate to embellish, add to or subtract from any of the
material presented. Make them your own.

You'll find here that a private practice is only limited by the limits
that we clamp around our imagination, and implementation!

A professional private practice is more than a place where we see
patients! Observe . . . .

Let Your Office Space Work For You

If you are in the position of having your own office and you have
space that is not being used, you may be able to make this open
space pay off. Determine how much space is not being used by you,
the hours available, and consider subletting the space out to other
therapists.

New private therapists typically get started by subletting office
space from someone who already has suitable facilities (see Chapter
2, p. 27). Your office space can be paying the rent while you are in
another office in the same suite working with patients. Or while you
are at home enjoying a steak dinner with your family, your office
can be paying for the meal!

Potential Subletters: Who is interested in subletting my office
space? Where do I find them and how do I let them know that the
office is open to them? The following target groups are good places
to begin advertising your office. A direct phone call or a "memo"-
type announcement are appropriate.

(1) Your local Psychological, Psychiatric, Marriage & Family
Counseling, and Social Work Association. These orgranizations
typically maintain a file of available office space open to subletters.
Ask them to list your office, give them location, hours available,
etc. Some may even list your announcement in their professional
newsletter or journal!

(2) The chairman of the local psychology, counseling, or social
work department at the university. Notice of your office availability
can be posted in a central place for faculty and/or students benefit.
NOTE: Should you be able to obtain all the names of the faculty
members in those departments, consider mailing each a brief
"memo"-type announcement of space available. You might mention
in their announcement that there are excellent hours open for part-

time, evening and weekend sessions, ideal for those who hold full-time jobs in teaching, etc.

(3) The chairman and individual therapists in psychology departments of local hospitals. (The annoucement memo is best).

(4) The administrator or individual counselors in local State and County Rehabilitation agencies, social work agencies, departments of probation and parole, adoption agencies, alcoholism and drug abuse treatment programs, etc. Your announcement will reach many individuals whose dream is to begin their own practice.

Office Availability Announcement: The flier, announcement, memo should be neat, brief and concise, detailing the advantages of your office for someone interested in seeing patients privately. Money, percentages or programs of payment should not be mentioned in the announcement. Figure 4 illustrates a typical memo announcement sent to staff psychologists at a local VA Hospital.

FIGURE 4. OFFICE AVAILABILITY ANNOUNCEMENT

PRIVATE PRACTICE OFFICE SPACE AVAILABLE

TO: All professionally licensed therapists (and interns) who are interested in part-time private practice.

SUBJECT: Professional office space now available to sublet.

Office Location: Office is centrally located near all public transportation. Less than 1/2 mile from two freeways. Modern suburban setting. Only 10 minutes from the University and VAH.

Description: Beautifully furnished modern office space in new professional building. Ample free parking. Air conditioned. Elevator service. 24-hour security service.

Hours Available: All weekday evenings. Tuesday and Thursday afternoons from 1 p.m. on. Saturdays all day.

Reasonable Rates.

FOR DETAILED INFORMATION, CALL DR. CHARLES BROWNING AT:

_____

Determining The Rental Rate: As we noted earlier, there are two commonly used means for setting the rate charged for the use of your office. You can employ the flat rate, or the percentage method.

Under the flat rate method, many therapists charge from $7 to $15 per hour for each hour used by the sub-tenant. This approach is recommended when (a) subletting to a new therapist who has very few patients; and (b) the therapist charges significantly below the going hourly fee.

The second method involves charging a percentage of the total fee charged by the subletter. This approach is preferable when (a) subletting to therapists with five (5) or more regularly scheduled patients; and (b) the therapist charges a competitive fee. The Southern California statistics range from 20% to 60% charged for gross patient fees, with a mean of 35%.

Tenant therapist typically collects rent once monthly. You may or may not ask subletter to specify number of hours in office, total patient fees collected, proportion, etc.

Use Of Secretarial & Answering Services: When subletting office space, it is common practice to offer the therapist the use of your secretary and/or answering service. You can do so at no additional charge, or you might follow the policy of charging an additional 5% for such services. Offering these services is especially attractive to the therapist just starting out. I do recommend, however, that caution be used here. If a therapist has several patients and intends moving into your office, the traffic on your phone and answering service may become a problem. Therefore, such a therapist would do well to provide his own answering service and telephone.

Patients Referred By You: Some therapists commonly refer patients to those who sublet from them. In such arrangements, some charge an additional 5% over and above the rent figure, or increase the hourly rate. This is optional, of course, and I am not recommending it.

Protect Yourself: Once you have made the decision to sublet to a therapist, get him to sign a sublet agreement. You want to be certain that you maintain a strict rental relationship with the therapist, and not a supervisory role. A sample Sublet Agreement is presented in Figure 5, (p. 108).

Professional Workshops

The workshop has become a popular tool by which many private therapists extend their service outside the consultation room. Both lay and professional audiences can be the target groups for work-

FIGURE 5. SUBLET AGREEMENT FORM

OFFICE SUBLET AGREEMENT

OFFICE PREMISES: 3662 Katella Avenue, Suite 214
Los Alamitos, California 90720

TENANT: Dr. Charles H. Browning

SUB-TENANT: _____

TERMS OF AGREEMENT TO SUBLET

A. 1. The above captioned parties enter into this agreement for purposes of providing professional office facilities for the practice of mental health services.

2. Tenant provides office space on a sublet arrangement to Sub-Tenant without any supervisory or clinical responsibility whatever.

3. Sub-Tenant is duly licensed to practice the specialty of ____, License Number _____ in the State of California. Or, Sub-Tenant is an intern working toward his own license under the supervision and license of _____ who assumes all professional responsibility for his work in the Premises.

4. Sub-Tenant is duly protected by professional liability insurance. Or, Sub-tenant is an intern who is protected by professional liability insurance of his supervisor, _____.

5. Tenant and owner assume no liability for accidental injury resulting on Premises.

6. Tenant agrees to assure proper maintenance and janitorial care of Premises.

7. Sub-tenant agrees to care for facilities in a careful manner with regard to safety, neatness, and cleanliness.

8. This agreement can be terminated by either Party with verbal notification at any time.

B. 1. Method of Rent Payment:_____
Date Due: _____

2. Designated Office Space for Sub-Tenant _____

3. Designated hours office Premises available to Sub-Tenant ____

4. Date Agreement Effective: _____

THE UNDERSIGNED AGREE TO ALL THE ABOVE CONDITIONS.

Date Signed _____

_____
Tenant

_____
Sub-Tenant

_____

shops on specialized subjects. Especially for the new independent therapist, the workshop can become an extremely effective practice builder. There are two important benefits in using the workshop to develop a healthy practice. (1) The income provided through the workshop can offset "dead time" in the practice. That is, time that no patients are scheduled — and in the early going, there is much of this. (2) Since the workshop reaches so many individuals, lay and professional, the therapist's practice gains new recognition. The professional workshop typically results in a steady stream of referrals to the practice.

Workshop Topic Material: Some of the most successful workshops these days include the following: (a) Assertive Training (and Assertive Training for Women); (b) Training for Effective Parenting; (c) Crisis Intervention Counseling; (d) Sexual Dysfunction Therapy; (e) Transactional Analysis; (f) Habit Control Thru The Use of Hypnosis; (g) Self Hypnosis Training; (h) Psychodrama and Sociodrama; (i) Marriage Enrichment and Marriage Encounter; and (j) Biofeedback Training. Workshop topics should be those in which you are highly trained and qualified. Subject matter should be practical, should include much member participation, and should be soundly grounded on reliable research data.

Promoting the Workshop: The most effective means by which to advertise your workshop is by means of an attractive brochure. You can prepare and distribute them yourself, at your own cost (and with the price of printing and postage stamps these days, that's not a small sum). Or, you can enlist the sponsorship of a local university. Many colleges and universities are now joining private professionals in holding workshops in mental health modalities. You might discuss your proposed workshop with the head of a counseling related department at the local university and propose joint participation. The school will assume the bulk of the financial arrangements. And if your topic has wide-spread public appeal, many radio stations and newspapers advertise such events as public service information *at no cost* to you! Send a short "blurb sheet" announcement to the program director or editor at least one month in advance of your workshop.

Broad-Spectrum Treatment Modalities

Some therapists in independent practice round out and broaden the impact of their work by offering to selected patients the opportunity to become involved in clinical experiences other than their one-to-one psychotherapy. Group therapy, conjoint marriage counseling, couple groups, weekend marathons (although these are of questionable clinical value), relaxation training, biofeedback training, and psychodrama and sociodrama make up just a few of those activities which can enhance the treatment process and the practice itself.

Some therapists are not comfortable in or qualified for such modalities. They therefore hire other professionals who are well versed in these approaches and supply both the facilities and the patients to them. The therapist may either directly supervise his work, or hire him as a consultant. If you should be interested in expanding your practice in this manner and need expert consultant help, a good place to find such assistance lies in the local graduate schools of counseling and psychology. Expert professional assistance at reasonable rates is available in this manner. *A practice need not be limited to those skills of the therapist himself.* Delegating treatment modalities to others can greatly increase the growth of a practice, and renders a valuable service to the community.

Social Security Specialist (Vocational Expert)

If you have training and experience in the areas of educational psychology, special education, rehabilitation counseling, or specialized work with the disabled, you may qualify for a federal consultant position. The Social Security Administration employs private therapists as Vocational Experts. The Vocational Expert reviews and analyzes appeal cases under the disability insurance program and makes court recommendations. The pay is good and it is a good source of funds to augment practice income. Space here does not permit an in depth explanation of application procedures, etc. If you are qualified and interested, write to:

Administrator
Vocational Consultant Program
Social Security Administration
P.O. Box 2518
Washington, D.C. 20013

Finding Office Personnel

When you find yourself ready to hire a secretary, file clerk, typist, or even a skilled therapist to see patients for you in your practice, don't forget the disabled! The State Department of Vocational Rehabilitation can very likely fill any need you may have for personnel with competent, reliable and highly motivated individuals. In some cases they will agree to an on-the-job training situation in which the agency pays you to train and perhaps hire the person. Contact the district administrator, State Department of Rehabilitation in your city.

Setting Up Industrial Mental Health Programs

Today more than ever before industry is recognizing its responsibility to deal with the mental health needs of its work force. The money is available in many companies for mental health services, but the know-how is lacking. Your experience and training could fill their need.

One therapist we know began his own practice and during those free hours he visited various companies in the city with a proposal. He had a great deal of know-how in the area of alcoholism treatment. He proposed that the company hire him as an outside consultant to set up an in-house alcoholism treatment program. He would assume responsibility for planning, hiring of staff, promoting the program to management and to employees, and when it was running smoothly, he would turn it over to management and personnel. His proposal was accepted by several good-sized firms in Southern California. The idea has grown so large that he had to turn his practice over to colleagues and he now devotes full time to setting up in-house alcoholism treatment programs.

If you can demonstrate to company management that your program would result in increased productivity, reduced absenteeism, improved personnel relations, and reduced employee attrition, you may find many interested customers.

Some companies are now becoming interested in the biofeedback training systems. If you have any expertise in this area, consider proposing a program to industry. In approaching companies remember: (1) Research the company well before approaching them; (2) Prepare a detailed, step-by-step proposal, and be *specific;* (3) Assume most of the responsibility for all phases of the program yourself; (4) Stress the advantages of cost savings and confidentiality of the in-house program; and (5) always begin at the top — i.e., propose the program first to the president of the corporation, then work down!

Industrial Consultation

Another good way to supplement fee income is by providing industrial consultation. Private industry hires private therapists as consultants in such areas as: behavioral analysis, employee-management relations, alcoholism treatment and diagnoses, leadership training, relaxation training, biofeedback training, human relations training, and so on. Some private therapists who are skilled in psychological testing are hired by personnel departments on a part time basis.

As we indicated above, remember to be knowledgeable about the company before approaching them, be specific in your proposal, tailor-make the service you offer to their need, and begin at the "top," or highest level of management. And be prepared to foot the bill for a lunch or two in negotiating the consultation position.

Biofeedback Training

It's too early to know whether biofeedback is here to stay, or whether it is another "psycho-fad." But the experiential and experimental evidence thus far looks promising. It may have good potential in private practice.

One therapist in a very successful practice uses biofeedback in conjunction with his individual counseling work. His secretary ushers the patient into the biofeedback room, hooks him or her up to the machines, and leaves the patient to his own therapy work with the machine for a period of time. This is a separate session to his regularly scheduled one-to-one session with the therapist. The therapist typically spends approximately ten minutes with the patient following each biofeedback session to examine results.

Like psychological testing, this may prove to be a useful adjunct to one's private practice, if the therapist is well trained himself in the use of such procedures. And in addition to clinical use in the office itself, don't overlook the potential for institutional use. You might consider proposing the development of a "biofeedback department" in industry, hospitals, schools, correctional institutions, convalescent homes, rehabilitation centers, etc.

Hot Lines & Emergency Telephone Services

Hot Line and Suicide Prevention Services are established to provide immediate help for crisis situations. Most of these services are not prepared to continue ongoing therapy with their callers. They rely on a pool of professional therapists in private practice and public agencies to follow through with the callers. In building your practice consider offering your services to the hot lines in your community. Most of them will be pleased to list you free of charge in their resource directory.

What about working for the hot line yourself? Volunteering your skills for a few hours a week can be wonderfully rewarding to you. As was noted earlier, GIVING AWAY your time and energy is the most powerful means by which you can accelerate the growth of your practice while serving your community (see pp. 50-51, "The Seed Principle: The Secret of A Dynamic Private Practice").

Does your area have adequate emergency hot lines and suicide prevention services? If not, why not organize such services yourself and provide the impetus necessary to implement it? Most hot lines are manned almost entirely by volunteers. A central answering service is used and workers take calls in their own homes. You might train lay volunteers in crisis intervention and hire the answering service at your own cost. You will find that referrals to your own practice will soon offset your investment. And most community media will advertise your service free of charge as public service information.

One innovative therapist on the East coast began a hot line called "TOT LINE." TOT LINE is a specialized hot line serving parents who have problems with child abuse and impulsive behavior toward their children. This idea has met with great success. Take a few moments here and consider this suggestion in light of the special needs in your own neighborhood. Could your community profit from emergency hot line services for alcoholics? For drug addicts? For those passing through the valley of a grief reaction? For the newly divorced person? For the LONELY? For the girl in conflict about whether to have an abortion? For the rape victim? For the elderly? For the runaway child?

The potential and impact of your practice is incredible and exciting!

Self-Help Training Tapes

A quick glance at the Classified section of most professional association newsletters and journals reveals that cassette self-help training tapes are on the increase — and are very popular. Relaxation training, assertive training, desensitization, guided imagery conditioning, speech therapy, cognitive behavioral conditioning, insomnia and depression aids, and the like are all being used professionally as adjuncts to traditional treatment.

Is your clinical work adaptable to audio-tape administration? You can reach thousands of people who, for whatever reason, may be unable to profit from in-office professional help, but who could receive help via a cassette tape. You can share innovative techniques with colleagues by way of taped demonstrations of your work.

Cassettes that you market should be of professional quality and should reflect the highest professional ethical standards (see Chapter 3). Any tape offered the public either for the training or treatment of any condition should always include in the presentation something along these lines:

> "The material contained on this recorded message should be used in conjunction with professional medical and psychological care. It is not intended to substitute for direct professional help."

Personnel Assessment Consultation

One Beverly Hills psychologist spends a part of his practice hours consulting with industry. Most of his work involves assessment of new applicants for sales positions for large insurance companies. These companies find a serious problem in reliability and longevity among new salesmen due to alcoholism or marital problems. The psychologist is hired as a consultant to evaluate each new applicant's probability for successful employment. He administers personality inventories, projective tests, simulated stress interviews, role rehearsals, and in some cases, consults with the spouse.

Should you have experience in testing and evaluation, consider this as a possible side-light to your private work. The rate of pay for industrial consultation is excellent. And as we noted in other areas of consultant activities, be sure to approach any company with (1) step-by-step, detailed proposals; and (2) a working knowledge of the company and its needs.

On-Site Behavioral Evaluations

School Evaluations: A friend in private practice recently began a new service in his practice. He hired an ex-school teacher who was well versed in behavioral analysis methods. She was sent to various schools to perform an in-depth behavior analysis for the children that the therapist was treating. The parents were eager to give their written consent to obtain such unusual information. Invaluable diagnostic and treatment data has been gathered by these on-site visits to classrooms, playgrounds, and visits with teachers and counselors in the schools. Regarding financial considerations, the parents are charged $75 for each visit to the school. This therapist has also sent out letters to other professionals in the area offering her services for their patients. The idea has much promise indeed.

Special Education Evaluations: One Southern California school psychologist began his first private practice after his retirement from the school district. Most of his work is spent testing emotionally and mentally handicapped children for their suitability for special education classes in the public schools. Under the "Sedgwick Fund", private practitioners are hired (and paid by parents of the children) to test and recommend the handicapped child for the best educational program.

Intake Test Batteries

Regardless of your orientation therapeutically, have you seriously considered the benefits of making psychological testing a part of your regular intake procedure with every patient? The advantages include the following for your practice: (1) Accurate clinical data can be gathered quickly and efficiently and much diagnostic time is saved; (2) The patient is smoothly and rapidly involved in the therapeutic process of self-disclosure through a non-threatening modality; (3) Through such involvement the patient is motivated to continue in therapy; (4) Clinical progress can more accurately be assessed; (5) The therapist is provided with "hard" data useful in the preparation of future research reporting.

Typical fees charged for test batteries range from 2 to 3 times the normal session fee rate. Should this idea appeal to you and find a place in your practice, and if you are one of those who knows little about the art and science of testing, consider this. Investigate hiring a graduate student in psychology or educational psychology to provide the expertise in testing your patients. While you are seeing other patients, he or she can perform the testing duties and prepare the reports. Do you remember how students (especially graduate students) need extra money? Experiment with the intake test battery for a month or so. You may be pleasantly surprised with the multi-faceted benefits to your practice!

Research Grant Funding

If you are now over the chronic writer's cramp which you endured during dissertation preparation, and should you enjoy conducting research and have a good track record of publications, this may interest you. A private practice can become an excellent vehicle for obtaining grant funding for mental health research.

The first step in making a private practice eligible for grant monies involves incorporating the practice. Most granting institutions (e.g., National Institute of Mental Health, National Institutes of Health, National Science Foundation, etc.) make it a policy to grant funds to non-profit organizations before considering private groups or agencies. How does one incorporate his practice and become a non-profit organization? The process is not a simple one, neither is it inexpensive! Before consulting an attorney, let me refer you to a book which can help save time, money and endless legal gymnastics. The book is entitled, "How To Form Your Own Corporation Without A Lawyer" by Ted Nicholas and can be ordered through the mail at $8.40 by writing to: Enterprise Publishing Co., 1000 Oakfield Lane, Wilmington, Delaware 19810.

With respect to the nuts and bolts of grantsmanship, let me recommend one further book to you. It's entitled, "The Applicant's Guide To Successful Grantsmanship" by Louis E. Masterman. This exhaustive guidebook can be ordered at $14.95 from: Keene Publications, 726 Watkins Drive, Cape Girardeau, Missouri 63701.

Approval for non-profit status for your practice takes some time. You can begin to utilize that time interval constructively by

(1) beginning initial work-ups on your grant proposal, (2) arranging for professional associates to assist you in the project (such as colleagues at local universities who may have access to a computer), and (3) begin writing letters and making phone calls to key personnel at the funding agency or foundation (get to know those instrumental in the grant process — you will learn to short-cut the red tape, and may develop a contact that could make the difference between acceptance or rejection of your proposal!).

And finally, one word of caution. When incorporating your practice as a non-profit activity, only those monies that come under the research classification are subject to this tax status. Other patient fees, consultation work, and so forth are not to be brought under the non-profit umbrella.

Supervision of Interns

When your practice reaches the happy point wherein the rate of referrals exceeds the number of hours open in your appointment book, consider supervision as a means to meet the growing demand for your work. Rather than referring patients out to another therapist, why not bring in a clinical intern?

There may be times when you do not choose to be in the office, for instance, during evenings or weekends. Those who are in graduate training or who are seeking clinical hours toward their licenses may be eager to fill those hours under your supervision.

The intern or assistant is typically paid a set hourly wage (e.g., anywhere from $5 to $25 per hour, depending on his or her experience).* You must meet with those under your supervision at least once weekly, and most states require that their work be conducted out of your office. It is also good practice to make monthly entries in their charts regarding your supervision.

Supervision of an assistant intern has many things to recommend it. While you build your practice, you are also sharpening your own clinical skills. There's something about teaching and supervision that keeps us on our toes clinically. And while the intern is seeing patients for you, you can have more quality time to spend with your family!

*The policy of paying interns nothing because of their need for earned hours is discouraged—Remember you get what you pay for, and what you don't!

Thesis & Dissertation Supervision

Some private therapists use free hours to provide consultation to graduate students. If you are skilled in research design, statistical analyses, generating original ideas for research worthy of publication, or editing and writing skills for publication, you may be in great demand. Due to the heavy burden on committee members, many graduate students seek outside help in their thesis or dissertation work. Let those faculty members at the counseling and psychology departments of your local universities know of your availability, specialty, rates, etc. Most committee chairmen will be overjoyed to let someone else get their shoulder under the weight of dissertation and thesis supervision! Your fee should be reasonable (perhaps $15 to $25 per hour).

Clinical Consultation To Private Schools

Private schools are growing at a tremendous rate. Unlike public schools, however, most private schools still do not have on-staff psychological or counseling personnel. Why not consider as a part of your practice a service providing on-site counseling and consulting services to private educational facilities?

You might propose to various private schools that you (or your clinical staff) visit the school on two or three half days each week. During this time, you could provide direct counseling services to students, students and parents, or to teachers and students together. Programs for in-service training for teachers might also be proposed in areas of behavior management or some specialized area within your sphere of competence.

This approach has particular value to the newcomer to private practice. It is a fine means to provide extra income while building your session hours. In planning to present this program to local private schools, prepare an attractive brochure and follow up mailings with a personal phone call and/or personal visit to the school director or principal.

This approach is so new (at least to the author) that no information can be reported here as to success or failure in the mental health area. However, other professionals have entered the private school "market" and have had overwhelming success. One group of nurses got together and offered their services in nursing instruction and patient care to private convalescent homes. Their business is thriving! Another small group of ex-school teachers combined to form a company in which they go from school to school offering courses in art, drama, music, tumbling, photography, etc. Their program has grown and doubled every year!

Explore the possibility of bringing mental health services to private schools via your own practice. And then let us know of your success so that we can report it in later editions of this handbook.

Pre-Paid HMO-Type Mental Health Plans

Perhaps the most exciting, and certainly the most lucrative idea to find success in private psychotherapy practice is the development of pre-paid mental health plans.

What is the pre-paid plan and how does it function? In a feature article (July 24, 1977) the *Los Angeles Times* reported the growing interest in pre-paid health programs, and gave this simple definition of how they work.

> "A prepaid group practice health plan charges a flat monthly premium for each member, regardless of how much or how little care the member receives. A doctor who works for a prepaid plan receives the same pay whether he delivers one or 10 services a day."

Pre-paid medical health plans have proved so successful in industry that Congress passed legislation to encourage the development of what they call Health Maintenance Organizations (HMO's). More recently here in California the idea has been proven extremely successful in the area of mental health services provided to industry.

Basically, this is how the program works. A group of professional people get together to join forces to provide comprehensive mental health services. The range of services from psychological testing, medical evaluation, individual and group therapy, marital counseling and family therapy comprise the group's "package." The group then makes a proposal to industry, offering to provide unlimited mental health services to all employees at a flat monthly rate. The employee pays in a minimal amount monthly through his union dues under his health coverage. The group is paid directly by the company on a per-capita basis; that is, a designated amount per employee. That amount is received whether two or twenty patients come for treatment. It is not difficult to see the potential of such a program!

At first glance it may seem that this approach has little application to a small private practice. But remember: Most group practices began with one or two professionals uniting themselves together to better serve the community. Any private practice with a well-balanced staff can offer pre-paid services to local companies. Even if you are a one-man (or one-woman) practice, you can successfully organize a pre-paid program to accelerate the financial growth of your practice.

You may be asking yourself at this point; "Is such a far reaching idea really possible in a small practice like mine?" The answer is absolutely, yes! "Do I have to have an existing 'clinic' and group of professionals to offer such services to industry?" Answer — No, not at all. From a one-person practice you can offer the same services that a huge clinic operation provides.

If the idea intrigues you (and it should because it is the most dynamic way to build a practice), here is one proven method to establish a successful pre-paid program through your own practice.

Step 1: Organize a panel of qualified therapists. Set about bringing together several licensed and competent mental health professionals in whom you have confidence. Seek to combine those professionals who will make up a well-balanced and comprehensive treatment team. For example, a psychiatrist, a clinical and/or counseling psychologist, marriage counselor, clinical social workers, and perhaps a certified rehabilitation counselor. Those professionals can be in their own practices, or have agency jobs. Ask them if they would consider becoming members of a treatment "panel" that you are forming for a pre-paid mental health program that you are developing. Tell them that you will assume responsibility for their fees for patients that you refer (NOTE: You are able to pay them out of the monthly premiums that you receive form the patient's employer).

Most professionals are interested in building their practices, or finding some outside private work, and you will find this step quite simple and direct. Once you have succeeded in enlisting these professionals as part of your panel, your comprehensive mental health group is formed!

It is not necessary that all the members of your group be housed under the same roof. As a matter of fact, it is much to your advantage to have them spread out over the community in their own offices. This has greater appeal to industry, whose employees may live in widely spread out areas. You become able to provide more accessible services through these "satellite offices." The clinic-type, one-office group cannot offer such benefits!

Step 2: You will need a practice name. In presenting your group to industry it will help to have a formal name. This is known as a "fictitious name" or "DBA" — "Doing Business As" label for your practice. In Chapter 9 we will deal with the particulars in forming the DBA (see pp. 126-128).

Step 3: Enlist the services of an insurance broker. Unless you are unusually skilled in the area of public relations, industrial relations, and the delicate art of working with union leadership, you'll need some expert assistance. An insurance broker is the man to call. Contact brokers who advertise in the Yellow Pages as handling Employee Benefits and Organization Plans. Inform him generally that you represent a group of mental health professionals, that you are now able to offer comprehensive, diversified and geographically strategic mental health services to industry, and that you are interested in hiring a broker that has some experience in pre-paid health plans. Ask him if he believes that he can handle the job.*

His responsibility includes finding those companies that may be interested in a pre-paid contract for mental health services in addition to other health benefits for their employees. He then will bring you and the management or leadership of the company together. The broker is simply a middle-man and your agent to "sell" your program to the company. What is his incentive, and how is he paid? The insurance broker works on a commission basis. Offer to give him a designated percentage (from 5% to 10%) of all contracts which he brings to the group and which result in successful closure.

It was noted in the outset of this chapter that "a private practice is more than a place to see patients." The pre-paid mental health concept is but one example to demonstrate the power, possibilities, and the potential of a private therapy practice. The only limits to this method of practice development are those you accept or create! This approach simply requires that you use some creative thinking, good planning and management of people, employ the best broker that you can find, and most importantly, that you enlarge your concept of private practice, and *aim high!** †

And one final requirement remains to make this, or any of the methods in this chapter, succeed for you. To succeed the particular method must be implemented, put into action. *ACTION!*

Which of the ideas in this chapter will *you* put into ACTION in your own practice during the coming week? Why not pause here, before continuing on to the next chapter, to plan your personal method of implementation?

Remember . . . *SUCCESS = TRUTH ACTED UPON!*

---

*Because of the changing legal conditions affecting the HMO corporate requirements, you are advised to consult a good corporation attorney on this one! Big Brother is making it increasingly difficult to get an HMO status.

† A complete legal agreement (contract) actually used to set up an HMO-type Employee Assistance Mental Health Program is available from Duncliff's. Ask for HMO/EAP—Contract, price: $5.

CHAPTER NINE

THE "WHAT IF'S" AND THE "HOW TO'S" OF A SUCCESSFUL PRIVATE PRACTICE

CHAPTER 9
THE "WHAT IF'S" AND THE "HOW TO'S"
OF A SUCCESSFUL PRIVATE PRACTICE

Questions and Answers

There are certain questions that this manual will *not* answer for you. For instance. In this manual you will not find detailed procedures for private practice bookkeeping and accounting. We'll leave that to a competent CPA (Certified Public Accountant). You will also notice that we pass over the matter of taxes, tax shelters, retirement plans, estimated tax payments, and other matters concerning Uncle Sam. Anyone serious about private practice should secure the services of a respected CPA who will not only answer all your tax and bookkeeping questions, but who will tailor make a program to best fit your needs.

Matters of legal concern to the independent therapist are also largely delegated to other professionals. We shall touch on the matter of how to prepare for court appearances on behalf of, or as professional witnesses for, patients, but matters of professional liability and suits and other legal issues are deleted purposely. When these questions come up the only best advice is to retain the services of a reputable attorney. And happily, you should rarely, if ever, require the services of legal counsel as part of your private work!

You should give careful thought to matters of hospital and medical insurance, disability insurance, retirement planning, and professional liability insurance. We recommend that you seek such information first through your professional association before consulting your local insurance agent. Again, we'll leave the details to others to give you the best data to suit your needs.

The last area that we omit in this manual, and that by design, is that of time management. This is a vital area to every person engaged in private practice in a part or full-time basis. Many clinicians are accustomed to someone else organizing their time, scheduling patients for them, and taking care of the paper work involved in administration. But in your own practice, "the buck stops at your desk." Space here does not permit a detailed exposition on time management and organization. Let me simply recommend a little book that could greatly help you get the most out of each hour. It's an invaluable aid to someone new to the business of self-employment. It's entitled, *How To Get Control of Your Time and Your Life,* by Alan Lakein, Signet, 1973.

Another book which provides some useful material on bookkeeping, legal aspects and general mechanics in a private practice is the following: *Practical Problems of a Private Psychotherapy Practice,* by Goldman and Striker, Charles C. Thomas, 1972.

Now that we have said what we shall not cover in this present chapter, let's see what we will cover together.

I have written this chapter especially with the newcomer in mind. Therefore, many of you old-timers may want to skim some of this material.

If it were possible for you and I to sit down together and discuss all the "what if's" and "how to's" about everyday issues in private work in psychotherapy I would want to give you a certain kind of answer. I would want to stay away from the abstract, the theoretical, or the idealistic. To help you succeed in your own practice (which is my greatest aim in writing this handbook) I must give you concrete, ultra-practical answers to your questions. So that is exactly what we shall do here.

I will provide "hard" answers to the most commonly asked questions, trying to anticipate many of those on your mind right now. The answers are intended to put your mind at rest, and direct you toward constructive, positive action leading to success in initiating or expanding your own practice.

But please remember . . . The responses to these questions are largely subjective in nature. They reflect the fruits of our own (and many others') trial-and-error, practice-makes-perfect experience. I have no empirical data to offer you, just the sincerest personal assurance that, "they get results . . . *they work!*"

So let's sit down together right now and have a cup of coffee and share some ideas together.

Q: What exactly is a "Fictitious Name" or "DBA" for a private practice? And is it necessary for me to have a DBA?

A: The letters "DBA" stand for "Doing Business As." It represents a name or title for a business enterprise. Sears, General Motors, The Community Counseling Clinic — all are DBA's. The DBA is also known as a "Fictitious Name." Most commercial businesses use fictitious names and many professional groups do also. *Psychological Affiliates, Center for Behavior Therapy, Southside Medical Group*—these are just samples of groups who have chosen to identify their practice with a title.

Whether you should use a DBA for your own practice, whether you are a one-man practice, or a group, I cannot conclusively answer for you. This is a very personal decision. But let me point out some definite advantages in doing so. First of all, using a DBA may increase your rate of referrals. Many patients when searching out a therapist in the "Yellow Pages" will call a "group type" DBA (e.g., *Counseling Associates*) before they would an individual therapist. Why? Apparently it is because they are more easily able to trust an institution before they can an individual. It's perhaps due to the same motives that cause me to prefer "Sambo's" over "Sam's Cafe!"

Secondly, if you plan to grow in your practice, a DBA is a good idea. If you have purchased this manual and have implemented any of the suggested approaches you are likely to see rapid growth in your practice. Even if you are alone at the outset, select a DBA that can *grow with you.* Ask yourself, "What would I call myself if I had a staff of five to ten therapists and had several satellite clinics under my supervision?" If you have absolutely no ambition to expand, then simply use your name and degree to represent your work. But if you are looking ahead with a vision, a Fictitious Name may be in order in your practice.

Thirdly, the formal DBA for a practice is advisable for those therapists who hope to receive referrals from governmental agencies. Community organizations will often refer patients to a "Center" or "Group" or "Institute" before they will refer to a one-man practice.

A fourth reason to select a Fictitious Name is that it is preferred by those individuals who may be seeking an internship placement while working toward their licenses.

And finally, if you intend to pursue the notion of a pre-paid mental health program through your practice, a DBA is a must!

To obtain a DBA for your practice, simply decide on the name and get in touch with your local newspaper. They will publish it in the legal notices section for you to make it legal. NOTE: When planning your practice name, be sure to observe certain legal restrictions, including: (1) has someone else previously chosen this name? (2) does my county or state permit such a title in my profession, i.e., to use the title "Clinic," "Center," or "Institute?" Some communities forbid certain labels unless the practice is incorporated, or has a specified number of employees on staff. Research this carefully!

So then. My personal recommendation to anyone who is moving into private practice with an attitude toward expansion, is this: Give your practice a "handle", an umbrella title that will fit your work and grow with you as you grow.

Q: What are some of the important administrative considerations for the newcomer to private practice?

A: Unlike some professionals (e.g., dentists, physicians) the psychotherapist or counselor can begin practice "on a shoestring." He need not purchase or lease expensive equipment. But there are a few items that you will need right away.

First of all, you will need to obtain professional business cards. They should be professional, simple and in good taste. For example, the card should be imprinted with your name, highest degree, specialty, and practice name if you choose. Office address and phone number should also appear. Many therapists imprint in the upper corner the phrase, "Office Hours By Appointment." It is a good practice to keep a supply of business cards (1) in the waiting room, (2) in the consultation room near the patient's chair or sofa, and (3) always handy in your own pocket or purse. You will be surprised at the rate the cards disappear in the waiting room and find their way into the hands of family and friends of patients!

Stationery and envelopes is the next item of inventory to consider. There are two ways you can approach this matter. You may simply have a printer print 500 or more letterheads and envelopes. This is not inexpensive. If budget matters are of concern to you at this phase, try this. Have a local stationery store make a rubber stamp for you containing your name, practice DBA, and address. Then you can use this to imprint envelopes and bond paper to serve as a letterhead. It may not be as attractive as the formal letterhead and imprinted envelope, but it will serve the purpose until your first few patients arrive!

Thirdly, there is the matter of the *business license*. Check with City Hall to see what the procedure is for obtaining your own business license. In most cities, even if you are subletting you will be required by law to purchase this license. They range in cost from $10 to $150 per year.

Q: Do you have any tips on office layout and furnishings?

A: If you are subletting office space this will be a matter of future concern to you. Should you have your own office, consider these ideas.

When selecting furnishings for the new office, choose them with an eye toward expansion and growth of the practice. You may be tempted at first to select somewhat inexpensive, "bare minimum" fixtures. Resist the temptation! We have found time and time again that patients and other professionals take note of the quality and comfort of furniture, the pictures on the walls, and the interior decor. Although the initial outlay of capitol may seem staggering at first glance (and it certainly did to us!), remember that it is all tax deductible!

When planning to furnish your office, you might ask yourself these questions: "Does this furniture, these wall hangings, lamps, etc., give the appearance of a thriving, successful professional practice?" "Are they comfortable?" "Do they create a soothing and tranquil place in which to wait or work?" "Are those furnishings in the office a good reflection of my own personality?"

Furnish the office with the patient always in mind. And use the visual and auditory stimuli to create a therapeutic "set", minimizing distractions, maximizing comfort. And purchase furnishings *as if* the practice were booming (even if the appointment book is empty!).

Q: How important is the layout of the waiting room?

A: Someone has said that treatment begins in the waiting room. Over a period of months the patient spends much time in your waiting room, perhaps time equivalent to several session hours! This time can be utilized for therapeutic purposes. The visual and auditory input can be chosen to prepare the patient for the work that he or she will enter in to on the other side of the consultation room door. The waiting room is much like the introduction to a good book!

Here are a few suggestions for your consideration.

Because of the nature of the work, individual chairs should be preferred to sofas or love seats. The waiting room should seat comfortably *more* people than would typically come for the largest group session, if space permits.

Live plants, ferns and flowers add much warmth and "life" to the office. Fishtanks or aquariums have a calming and relaxing effect. Pictures of landscapes or seascapes bring about a serene and peaceful set for waiting patients.

Many therapists provide coffee and other drinks for patient use. Instant coffee, creamer, Tang, tea, and cocoa can all be kept accessible to patients either in the waiting room or in the consultation room.

Privacy is a must in the waiting room. Consultation rooms should have double doors, or the doors should be of solid construction with door sweeps and insulation. To further soundproof the waiting area from the therapy rooms some form of "white noise" should be present. Most office buildings provide piped-in music to act as white noise or background sound. If this is not the case in your building you can purchase white noise devices. Or you might create your own with pre-recorded tapes of your favorite music or "Environmental Sounds."

The selection of reading material in the waiting room is of utmost importance. It may not be an issue in the barber shop or the dentist's office, but it is in the psychotherapist's office! All material in the waiting room should be carefully chosen to ready the patient for the upcoming hour. Inspirational books such as *"Leaves of Gold"* are conducive to deepening patients' thoughts and settling them. Books that can be read in a few minutes, such as *The Giving Tree* and *The Missing Piece* by Silverstein provoke the patient to enter into contemplative patterns of thinking even before he or she sees you. High quality magazines such as *National Geographic* and other pictorial journals are good sources to settle and "set" the patient for therapy. *The Holy Bible*, Almanacs, and good humor magazines are to be preferred over the newsstand woman's periodicals. *Every* item in the waiting room should be "planted" there, so to speak, to create in the patient an attitude of hope and positive expectancy toward the therapeutic hour.

If you're brave and like taking risks why not try this. Put a small bookcase in the waiting room. Place good inspirational and self-help books there that can be checked out and taken home by patients. Rubber-stamp your name and address and phone number all over the books and have patients check out books in a check out pad. Expect some of these materials to disappear from time to time, but hopefully it will be well used and will help someone through a dark period of their life.

For those patients who must bring their children with them, and for the "little patients," why not have a stack of coloring books, pads and crayons available? Some therapists have a toybox in the waiting room or in a separate play room.

Q: How can one effectively handle the initial telephone contact with a prospective patient?

A: Someone has said that the first five minutes of any relationship are the most important. That may be a bit extreme. But it does shed some light on the first phone contact with a potential patient.

That first encounter over the phone is more than just an appointment-scheduling ritual. The patient has made a most difficult decision — to share his most intimate life problems with a perfect stranger! He or she will have their "antennas" fully extended and will try (however subconsciously) to get a "reading" on you. "Can I trust this therapist? Is he sympathetic to my problem, or will he just treat me like a number? Will I be just a "patient" to him or a *person?* Will he be patient with me until I can learn to trust him? For the therapist this call may merely represent another slot occupied in his appointment book. For the caller, he or she may be going down for the third time and desperately crying out for a life line.

During the first contact, therefore, work at being as warm, compassionate and genuinely concerned as possible. Avoid coming across as coldly clinical or overly serious. Put the potential patient at ease by a smile in your voice. Keep in mind that trust and rapport are on the line during these few moments. Use them well!

Many therapists lose many would-be patients right here during their first meeting over the phone. A stuffy, clinical, sober attitude accounts for some of the attrition. And more are perhaps lost due to the therapist's lack of preparation in answering basic questions that will arise. Be ready to give the caller simple, plain and down-to-earth answers to such questions as the following:

What are your fees?

What about insurance?

How often will I have to come in for therapy?

Will I be seen alone? With my spouse? In a group?
What is your orientation? (training? background?)
Do you think you can help me with this problem?
How long will it take?

You will be asked most of these questions. Rehearse your responses.

Many first-time callers almost seem to slip into their first session over the phone. Unless you are well structured and systematic during this initial contact, you may end up conducting your first session over the phone — for free!

To help you structure the initial phone screening interview, here is a sample outline (Figure 6) of an effective approach to minimize time loss. You might adapt the following to conform to your own personality and style.

FIGURE 6. **INITIAL TELEPHONE SCREENING FORMAT**

I.   Building the Relationship.

    A. Be friendly. Warm. Genuinely interested. Smile in my voice.

    B. Be positive. Give hope. Supportive.

    C. Re-label the presenting problem as "the current situation" or "the present difficulty." Do not label in terms of "the problem." (Helping the caller to begin redefining the problems in more positive terms begins the therapy process).

II. Gathering Data.

    A. Lead-in: "It's best, since our work together will be completely confidential, that we do not get into too much detail over the phone. So, if you would, just briefly give me an idea of some of the important information for now . . ."

    B. Who referred you to us?

    C. Does the current situation involve you alone, or are other members of your family also effected?

    D. Does the current difficulty involve any marital conflicts? Drugs? Hospitalization? Alcohol? Legal difficulties? Other?

III. Fees; Insurance Data.

    A. State fees, method for determining fee (if sliding scale), arrangement for payment (whether pay-at-time-of-consultation or method for billing).

    B. Ask about insurance coverage. Advise patient that claims are submitted monthly for his reimbursal. Ask patient to bring blank claim forms at time of first session.

    C. Get patient to agree on amount of fee and manner of payment.

IV. Preliminary Homework.

(Many therapists elect to assign pre-session homework in order to get the patient quickly involved in the therapy process, even before the first meeting. This is especially effective where an initial test battery is not employed. The method also works to overcome the patient getting "cold feet" [anticipatory anxiety] and failing to show for his first session).

A. Lead-in: "To help you organize your thinking for our first meeting together, and to help me to get a good understanding of the situation, I'd like for you to jot down some brief notes on some questions and bring it in (or mail it in) when you come. Do you have a pencil handy?"

(The following questions can be used, or you can send caller a detailed questionnaire of your own choosing).

B. Please describe any previous (or current) therapy? Who was (is) the therapist? When? For how long? Outcome?

C. Are any drugs being used now? In the past? Specify.

D. Has there been any suicidal ideas? Attempts? Plans?

E. Please describe the present difficulties in your own words.

F. How have you tried to deal with this situation? What has worked best for you up to this time? How are you handling it today?

G. Who are the people in your life most helpful to you in handling this difficulty?

H. What are your goals for our work in therapy together? What would you like to see happen in your life? Please be specific.

V. Set Up First Appointment.

Arrange for day and time of first session. Give office address with clear directions. If patient will find a waiting room with no receptionist, inform him or her of this fact. Some patients are unduly confused and additional stress is added when they fail to find the expected "doctor's office" receptionist. Plan for this and put them at ease at once. Endeavor to set up first session as soon as possible after first contact. If a week or more passes, the courage that moved him to call may melt away (or freeze over!).

Q: How should I handle "No-Shows?"

A. The "No-Show" is the ongoing patient who habitually fails to arrive for scheduled appointments without notice to therapist. A great deal can be learned about the patient by such behavior. When you find your waiting room empty when a patient should be occupying a chair there, spend some of the next hour asking yourself these probing questions:

What is the patient telling me about himself by this behavior?

What is he telling me about our relationship?

What is his absence telling me about ME?

You might then use the hour to go back over the chart notes to discern the answers. Time spent in this way will greatly enhance future work with this patient, and will sharpen your own clinical skills.

The patient himself should be gently and directly confronted with the issue of no-show during the next consultation. Sharing with him or her what you have discovered during your prior research (above) would be most effective and therapeutic.

Many therapists feel that the patient should be charged full fee if 24-hour notice is not given for cancellation. This is up to you. We do not use this procedure in our own practice, however. Personally, this method seems rather punitive and counter-therapeutic.

Here is one effective and novel means to handle the no-show. When the pattern becomes chronic, the therapist simply *prescribes the no-show*. That is, he takes hold of the problem, redefines it in a healthy way, and helps the patient avoid another failure experience. The patient is advised that the recent string of unattended sessions indicates that patient should experiment on his own, without therapy, for a time. A "vacation" from therapy is recommended. Using this approach, when the patient returns he or she is typically ready to assume more responsible behavior, with a renewed commitment.

Q: Is there any "best" length of session time in private practice?

A: This has always been a troublesome area for me personally. It's so easy to get caught up in the session and to forget that, "Time waits for no man." Result? With a full patient schedule, whenever one session runs overtime, all the sessions are disrupted. And at the end of the day you are late for dinner!

Solution? If you just cannot remember to look at your watch, use a timer.* Put a minute-timer in a desk drawer. Set it to ring (with a soft bell) 5 minutes prior to ending time of the session. This gives you ample time to summarize and reschedule. Some therapists position a fairly large wall clock immediately behind the patient's chair or sofa to help control the hour. Another idea is that of using a Westminster chime clock that chimes on the quarter hour in the consultation room. The atmosphere created is therapeutic, the ticking is quieting and relaxing, and the chimes are a perfect signal to end the session.

---

*The new electronic calculators enable you to set a small beeper-alarm to signal session end. The Texas Instruments "Data-Chron" is one of the best.

What is the "best" session length? This is like asking, "what is better, chocolate, vanilla, or strawberry?" Purely subjective. The 45-minute hour is becoming more and more popular these days among private practitioners. I suppose this could be justified if the practice has a lengthy waiting list with patients scheduled back-to-back all day long. But even then, the question remains: Does the 45-minute hour result in rapid and lasting change? Are we becoming more proficient in briefer psychotherapy? Or, are we becoming more mercenary? If you will recall, the secret to building a thriving practice is to GIVE more than is expected or required. In determining your session length as policy, keep that in mind. "It is in giving that we receive." (cf. "The Seed Principle: The Secret of a Dynamic Private Practice, pp. 50-51).

And in planning session length, remember to give yourself a few quiet moments between each session for charting, telephone messages, or R. and R.!

Q: In private practice is it absolutely necessary to keep charts?

A: If you come from a university or hospital setting you are likely up to your eyebrows in paper work. You would probably like to do away with all such work in your practice, including charting. Right? But, with the privilege of your own practice comes the responsibility. We are responsible to every patient to remain accountable. Charting helps you to keep informed on progress and guides you toward achieving therapeutic goals. Your records are subject to subpoena by any court (no more professional immunity! as evidenced in some recent court decisions against colleagues).

In addition to this, should you ever desire to conduct research in your practice, charting records are invaluable sources of data.

And as we noted in our discussion of generating referrals, the information in the chart can point the way to valuable contacts for practice growth; e.g., patients' physician, significant others, pastor, etc. A special place on the inside of each chart folder can be designated, "Patient Contacts" to help during your weekly practice review. Name, relationship to patient, date contacted and date of planned future contact can be entered here.

Q: How should I handle court appearances?

A: You may hear a knock on your office door one day and when you answer that knock you may find someone placing an official-looking paper in your hand. It's not the mail, it's a subpoena calling you to appear in court on behalf of one of your present or past patients. This calls for you to cancel an entire day's appointments and wait in the courtroom until you are called. What can you do?

(1) Contact the attorney immediately. Get him to agree to call you as an "expert witness" and not an "eye witness." What's the difference? The difference involves your being paid from $100 to $500 per day as compared to from $10 to $20 a day respectively!

(2) Should the attorney not agree to call you as an expert witness, try this. Gently inform him that in light of this, you would perhaps not be the most friendly witness and would have nothing positive to contribute to his case. This may induce him to cooperate for the sake of his cause.

(3) Since the attorney is the patient's agent, you may discuss the matter with the patient. Patient should be apprised that you are being asked to cancel the day's patients and would he be willing to finance or reimburse you? If not, have him instruct attorney to dismiss you.

(4) If you find yourself on the witness stand as an "eye witness" as soon as you are asked a professional opinion, ask to address the judge directly. Inform him that you have not been called as an expert witness and therefore cannot answer this question involving professional opinions. The judge may then reclassify you then and there. Then your fee will be met!

(5) Should you find yourself backed into a corner by an unfriendly lawyer while on the witness stand, turn to the judge and say, "Your Honor, may I qualify this response?"

(6) I claim no expertise in the legal arena, only some "what seems to work" practical advice. So when you find that subpoena in one hand, dial your attorney on the phone with the other! "In the multitude of counsellors there is safety."

Q: In my own practice is it necessary to have an Employer Identification Number?

A: According to IRS, you must obtain an Employer Identification Tax Number if "(you) paid wages of $1,500 or more in any calendar quarter, or (you) had one or more employees at any time in each of 20 calendar weeks . . ." (Circular E: Employer's Tax Guide, IRS, 1975).

So should you hire a receptionist, secretary, or counselor and the above criteria are met, you must have the number.

But even if you are a one-man (or woman) operation, we recommend you get the number anyway. Why bother? Simply because many insurance companies request this number on their claim forms. To assure more speedy reimbursement for your self and your patients, the number adds weight to the claim. "Our's is not to reason why . . . our's is just to play the game!"

You can apply for this number by writing to:

Department of the Treasury
Director, IRS Center
5045 E. Butler Avenue
Fresno, CA 93888

Q: When should the matter of fees be taken up with patient? Is there any "best" time?

A: If you will recall, in Figure 6, pp. 132-133, we outlined a sample phone screening procedure. It is during this first contact that the patient should be informed of his or her financial responsibility. If the matter of fees is discussed openly and candidly before the first session and the patient agrees to the fee and manner of payment, a kind of *verbal contract* has been established. So when the patient arrives for their first session they are confirming their intent to follow through. The issue of the fee then becomes a non-issue in the therapeutic process.

Q: As a clinician, I am somewhat uncomfortable in dealing with money matters in therapy. Is there any way to put both the patient and myself at ease and make the fee less of a sticky issue?

A: Awkwardness in dealing with money is a common complaint among clinicians. Largely because in the hospital or clinic setting others have acted as "shock absorbers" for them and collected the fees. Now the onus is on you! What to do?

Here are some helpful suggestions that may put you at ease, neutralize the $$$ issues, and will help to get on to the business of therapy.

(1) You will be more comfortable with the matter of fees if you have a definite fee schedule. You must decide whether you will

charge a flat fee to all patients, or use a "sliding scale" which is determined by patient's gross or net family income.

(2) As we already noted, fees should be discussed early on in the initial contact. You, or the patient can broach the subject. Try to maintain a self-assured, determined, and a matter-of-fact attitude when discussing fees.

(3) Patient should be told the amount of the fee, the time or length of session, whether individual, conjoint or group sessions are involved, the manner in which the fee is to be paid (monthly billing or payment at the time of session), and discuss whether patient has insurance that will reimburse him.

(4) Therapist should then get patient to commit himself or herself to the fee amount, to take responsibility to pay fee according to the plan just expressed, and to assure therapist that such fee will cause no undue financial hardship on patient.

To illustrate how one therapist smoothly and effectively handles the fee issue, observe this response to patient's question, "What is the charge for each session?"

THERAPIST: "You'll be seen individually and the session fee is $60. The session is approximately one hour in length and all patients pay their fee AT THE TIME OF CONSULTATION, at the end of each session. This eliminates the need for monthly billing and keeps your fees manageable.

Also, should you have any insurance that may cover your work in therapy, bring any claim forms with you at the time of the first session. We will submit them for you each month so that you can be reimbursed by the company.

Now, is this all suitable to you? It is important that you are comfortable with this fee and that it is acceptable to you. Is this clear to you? Are there any questions at all?"

Experience has shown that if the matter of fees is handled in such a forthright, easy-going, and direct way it soon becomes a dead issue. Incidentally, when patient is informed of the pay-as-you-go manner of payment as above we have never encountered any objection whatever. See pp. 141-144 for a more detailed discussion of this subject.

Q: What are the guidelines for establishing fees in private practice?

A: In their publication, "Ethical Standards of Psychologists" The American Psychological Association outlines three important considerations in setting rates in a professional practice.

"In establishing rates for professional services, the psychologist considers carefully both the ability of the client to meet the financial burden and the charges made by other professional persons engaged in comparable work. He is willing to contribute a portion of his services to work for which he receives little or no financial return."

(1) *Ability of the client.* The aim in private practice is to provide professional services to as many individuals in the community as require them. A system that adjusts to the financial condition of the patient is best. Many therapists use what is called the "sliding scale." Fee rate is determined by either the patient's gross or net family income. Figure 7 illustrates two sample sliding scale methods.

FIGURE 7. **SLIDING SCALES FOR INDIVIDUAL PSYCHOTHERAPY**

Sample Scale A

GROSS FAMILY INCOME		RATE PER HOUR*
From	To	
$20,000	& up	$60.00
$17,000	$19,999	$50.00
$15,000	$16,999	$40.00
$13,000	$14,999	$35.00
$11,000	$12,999	$30.00
$ 9,000	$10,999	$25.00
below $9,000		Negotiable**

Sample Scale B

NET FAMILY INCOME	RATE PER SESSION*
$20,000 & up	$70.00
1-2 dependents	$60.00
3 + dependents	$50.00
$18,000 to $20,000	$45.00
1-2 dependents	$45.00
3 + dependents	$40.00
$16,000 to $18,000	$40.00
1-2 dependents	$35.00
3 + dependents	$35.00
$14,000 to $16,000	$30.00
1-2 dependents	$30.00
3 + dependents	$25.00
$10,000 to $14,000	$20.00
below $10,000	Negotiable**

* Session hour ranges in length from 50 to 60 minutes.

** In exchange for professional services, patient agrees to donate his own time to those in need.

---

(2) *Charges by other professionals.* Before deciding on a fee schedule, take a random sample of therapists in your area. This will give you a "feel" for the fee climate in your community.

But one caution please. During the past few years there has been an unfortunate tendency in our profession to decrease the 50-minute hour to 45, and even to 30 minutes, and to increase the fee to $50, and $75 and even more per session. We see this trend in psychiatry, psychology, marriage counseling and in social work. For this reason, it is strongly recommended that more emphasis be placed on client ability to pay than on keeping pace with our colleagues. Even though you may be tempted to charge $60 per 45-minute hour in your practice because it's "common practice", consider the consequences. You will certainly earn more per hour. But you will, over time, spend far fewer hours with patients due to lack of referrals, a heavy drop out rate, and because you have chosen to place the emphasis on "getting" and not on "giving!" Keep the fee client-centered.

Down the hall, and at the other extreme, from the get-rich-quick clinician is the newcomer to private practice who feels that in order to build his practice he should charge practically nothing for his time. He may spend an hour and a half with each new patient and charge them a flat $20. Both the 45-$60 and the 90-$20 therapist are swinging toward the extreme ends of the continuum; and *extremes seldom prosper!*

Even though you may be new to your own practice, remember this. Those coming to you don't know that. They know that you have spent years in costly preparation and training for this work. They are accustomed to paying their physician, their dentist, their attorney a professional remuneration. So establish a fair, flexible and professional fee.

(3) *Little or no return.* My statements regarding the get-rich-quick, 45-$60 policy will be less than popular with some who read this manual. My next comment will likely appeal even less to this group. I've said it before, and here it is once more. The most effective way to insure rapid and dynamic growth in your practice is to GIVE AWAY a proportion of your time and skill. This is what APA daringly asserts in their Ethical Standards. How many therapists would you estimate follow this practice?

If you could survey those practices that are steadily growing and those that receive regular referrals from the community, other professionals, and from their own patients you would doubtless find the policy in practice. If you were to question those whose practices "just didn't seem to get off the ground," you would find the opposite. Practice growth and practitioner generosity are two sides of the same coin!

"As you sow, so shall you also reap!" The business community calls this principle "Good Will." I call it compassion. By any other name, it would still smell as sweet! And believe me fellow colleague, it is as practical as any principle or strategy in this book. In building your practice, *GIVE!*

One final point regarding sliding scales. It is a good idea to print your scale on a card and have it handy. You will need to refer to it when screening callers on the phone, to show to some patients in the office, and, should you have a secretary, for her to use as a guide to handling new patients.

If you will note in Figure 7 those patients who are seen at "No Charge" are asked to donate their time to the needy. This policy stimulates both responsibility and therapeutic gain in the patient with low income. We suggest such activities as making a weekly visit to a convalescent home to cheer a lonely old person; or to write a letter a week to someone whom they have felt bitterness toward; or to do one loving/unselfish thing per week for a parent; or to spend some time each week in volunteer work in a hospital or in their church. We have even urged some patients who could not afford therapy to spend an equal hour each week after their own session by calling lonely or depressed patients! "Payment" for these patients has far reaching implications!

Q: Is there any "best" method for the collection of fees?

A: A "best" method is the method that WORKS! You have a choice between several modes of collecting patient fees. You can bill the patient weekly, monthly, bi-monthly, or on some other interval basis. Or you can receive payment at the time of session. All of the above alternatives are employed by professionals in private practice. But which one WORKS?

Billing the patient, on whatever schedule, keeps the matter of money out of sight and eases the therapist's anxiety about collecting fees. But there are some serious drawbacks to billing.

If you would do a little research and ask other therapists how much money they have never collected, how much they carry in Accounts Receivable, you would likely find little difficulty in deciding on the method of choice.

Billing requires stationery, postage and time. It also brings with it a personal effect on the therapist . . . headaches! Many therapists who bill their patients carry thousands of dollars of "bad debts" on their books. Terminating therapy because of unpaid bills, or asking a collection agency to hound the money out of the patient, or taking legal action are destructive to the patient's emotional welfare, and should not be used in the mental health field, in my opinion.

What is the alternative? *Pay-at-the-time-of-consultation.* If this method is defined to patient at the outset, and if the patient is casually reminded of this at the end of the first session, the immediate payment policy is easily established. Commenting to the patient as you are entering his next appointment in the book, "Your next session is next Tuesday at 11 a.m., and this session is $60, do you need a receipt, or will it be a check?" is an effective way to remind the patient to get out their checkbook.

At first glance this method of collecting fees may seem a bit cold and mercenary. But in practice the "sting" is taken out of fee payment for the patient — it is easier on one's financial conscience to write out a check for $60 once weekly than to enter $240 in the checkbook monthly!

My advice to you? Eliminate accounts receivable. Eliminate billing. Eliminate headaches! Try the pay-as-you-go method and you will never regret it.

Q: Do you have any tips for handling the patient who "forgets" to pay as he goes?

A: Some patients will test your resolve to collect fees each week. Others will simply forget to leave the check. This can become an uncomfortable moment for both if one does not know how to respond to it well. Here are a few ideas that work nicely.

1. As noted above, remind patient as you enter his next appointment in the schedule book; "Do you need a receipt?"

2. If many patients are leaving and you are left without a check, it may indicate that you are a bit uneasy about communicating the policy to patient. If so, try this. Get a duplicate cash receipt book. Make it a habit to give *every* paying patient a copy of the receipt, whether they use check or cash. In this way at the end of every session the nonverbal cue of your making out the receipt signals patient to make out his check. Point out to patients that they should keep the receipts, as well as their cancelled checks, as their sessions are income tax deductible.

3. Humor is a good release during such a moment as this. If the above method fails, look squarely at the patient, smile, and say something like, "It's check time!"

Use whatever idea works best for you, or develop one of your own. But by all means be ready, be prepared for this situation to avoid awkward moments.

Q: If the patient is covered by an insurance program, is a pay-as-you-go procedure still recommended?

A: Although the patient may believe that he is covered by insurance for his therapy, often the company will pay part or none of the fee. The whole business of insurance reimbursal is so erratic and unpredictable that it is best for you to receive payment from patient, and let the company deal directly with patient for reimbursal.

Another reason to maintain the pay-as-you-go policy is that even if the insurance carrier pays the full fee, they often take from six to twenty weeks to reimburse.

Inform patient during first contact that you will submit his claim monthly and he will pay you at the time of consultation, while the company reimburses him directly. But if patient cannot bear this burden, be flexible; make exceptions.

Q: How should I deal with the issue of the patient who gets behind in his payments?

A: First of all, try not to allow the problem to go beyond two or at the most three sessions. If you come to the end of the session and patient has somehow forgotten his checkbook *again*, take this action. Advise the patient of the total amount due and ask that he or she send you a check for that amount *prior to the next session*. If check is not received by time of next session, therapist should deal gently—but firmly—with the issue at that time.

It is a good operating procedure to ask the patient who fails to pay even after one session to mail you the check prior to his next session. This works extremely well.

Q: In private practice should a patient be charged for time spent with him over the telephone between sessions?

A: Many patients become dependent on frequent contacts with the therapist and may put in frequent calls to you between sessions. Much that is therapeutic can be accomplished over the telephone. But if you are not careful, many hours may be spent in consultation with him or her at no remuneration to you whatever.

For this reason many therapists inform patient that time spent in consultation over the phone between regularly scheduled appointments will be billed for and, if possible, must be scheduled also. For example, early on in the screening process a patient may be informed as follows:

"I understand that you may need to talk with me from time to time between our regular sessions. And this is fine. In order for me to have sufficient time to spend with you, we must schedule any phone consultation time. The time spent in work on the phone will be charged at the regular rate and can be paid at the next office visit, along with the fee."

When the patient calls and requests time with you on the phone, patient should be advised to call you back at a set time which is entered in the appointment book. This implies the formality of the call and designates the time as consultation time. Note that the patient *calls you*. This is important due to message units and long distance rates that you should avoid, if possible.

The patient might be advised that until the time of his scheduled call he or she jot down notes to organize his or her thinking to get the most out of your time together on the phone.

This method may not be appropriate for every patient, or for every therapist for that matter. It is especially useful for the chronic caller who spends more time with you on the phone than they do in your office!

Q: Can regularly scheduled sessions be carried out entirely over the telephone?

A: Most of our work involves verbal communication and interaction, nonverbal skills notwithstanding. It has been our practice and experience that quality therapeutic work can be accomplished using the phone entirely, if necessary.

Telephone consultation has served as the mode of choice for a variety of reasons. Some patients are home-bound and because of some physical impairment are unable to come into the office. Others have work hours that conflict with the normal working hours of the therapist. Many patients have no means of transportation and can only avail themselves of your services over the phone. And some patients because of the "stigma" that they see in their involvement in therapy, "don't want to be caught dead coming out of a shrink's office!" The telephone solves the problem nicely.

Please note, however, that we are not recommending this method of psychotherapy over the face-to-face encounter with the patient. Telephone consultation is a "when all else fails" modality . . . and a most effective one!

Q: When my patients require medications, how does the non-MD therapist obtain psychiatric consultation for meds?

A: Sooner or later a patient will require psychiatric evaluation for medication. If you don't know a friendly psychiatrist you'll have to do some shopping around.

Ask colleagues if they could recommend a competent psychiatrist. Call this doctor and ask him if he "would be willing to see my patients occasionally, as needed, for medication evaluation." (And don't forget to tell him who referred you to him!) Most psychiatrists in private practice will be glad to get the referrals.

It is important that you DO NOT PROPOSE THAT HE BECOME YOUR PSYCHIATRIC CONSULTANT *per se.* If you propose such an arrangement, it may cost you an arm and a leg, and it isn't worth it. Simply propose to him that he see your patients for meds, evaluate and make disposition, and bill them directly. You will be responsible for their ongoing treatment. Assure him that in no way is he responsible or in supervision over your work. He'll just be handling medication follow-up.

Such a relationship with a psychiatrist may also prove valuable to you whenever psychiatric hospitalization is contemplated. And you may receive referrals through this contact (but don't hold your breath!)

Q: Do you have any tips on the selection and use of a good answering service?

A: Before answering this question, a word about answering machines. Although the telephone answering machines are much cheaper to maintain, there are serious problems in their use. Most people feel awkward and clumsy in talking to a tape recorder. Right from the first call the prospective patient should be put at ease as much as possible. For this reason alone, I would strongly urge you to use an answering service. They have their faults, as I am the first to attest, but at least they are warm bodies who can interact with the caller — *life touching life.*

Finding an efficient and reliable answering service is not easy. The girls are typically underpaid and overworked and under-trained. But to help you avoid some of the frustrations of the activity, here are some ideas.

(1) Before deciding on a particular service, shop around. Talk to colleagues. How would they rate their present service? Compare monthly rates, the amount charged per call, amount charged for messages relayed or ring-throughs to you?

(2) The service should offer 24-hour coverage for your office phone and should be familiar with professional, doctor-office accounts.

(3) When you have selected the service, prepare the following information on an index card for the operator to see at a glance:

    a) Your name, practice name, specialization.

    b) Your home phone number (not to be given out to callers).

    c) Hours you are in the office.

    d) On what ring phone should be answered by service.

    e) How phone should be answered; e.g., "Dr. Jones' Office" versus "Dr. Jones' Exchange" versus "Jones' Therapy Group."

    f) What to tell patient or caller when you are not available to talk; e.g., "Dr. Jones is with a patient now" or "I'm sorry, Dr. Jones is in consultation with a patient; he'll get back to you."

    g) What to do in case of an emergency; instructions to ring-thru to you in the office, or where to reach you after hours, etc.

    h) Emergency phone number should you be unavailable; e.g., a local hot line or suicide prevention center number.

    i) Specified time you call patients back. Some therapists set aside a specific hour each day (say, from 5 to 6 p.m.) at which time to return patients' calls.

    j) List associates who work in your office and how they may be reached.

(4) Some patients get upset when they try to reach you and get the girls on the answering service. The girls often take their share of verbal abuse and act as shock absorbers for you.

It's a good idea to coach the girls from time to time when a particular patient causes trouble for them. For example, you might say, "When Mrs. Smith calls, she may get a bit upset. Just listen patiently to her and tell her that I have told you to expect her call. Tell her that I will call her as soon as I am free. And I really appreciate your being patient and kind with her; you are helping me help her!" Or, "When Mr. Doe calls, please remind him gently that his next appointment is on Monday at 10 a.m. and that Dr. Jones would like for him to write down his thoughts right now and bring them in with him during his next session."

It is our responsibility to talk with any patients who continue to cause problems with the girls and to help patient handle the girls with more courtesy.

(5) *Call your answering service often!* When you call in and check on messages often the girls get to know you and in turn you will get better service. And in addition to calling the service on your special switchboard number for messages, call your own office phone number from time to time. In this way you can personally check to see whether they are answering quickly, efficiently and with warmth.

(6) Be friendly and courteous with the girls (but using your title and remaining professional). Get to know their names . . . and use them. But be careful. It has been our experience that becoming too friendly with the operators results in less efficient service. Find the happy balance.

(7) From time to time evaluate the service through your patients. Ask them how they are handled when they call in? How many times does the phone ring? This is a good quality control measure and should be done regularly. Perhaps you might schedule one week

every so often in which you ask all patients to comment on the service.

(8) When you are away, be sure to leave word with the exchange where you can be reached.

(9) A card or flowers or candy at Christmas time is a wonderful gift to repay their hard work for you . . . and the giving results in better service to your patients!

If there are other questions that I have neglected, I would be happy to deal with them in personal correspondence. Feel free to write!

CHAPTER TEN

THE CARE AND FEEDING OF A PRIVATE PRACTICE

CHAPTER 10
THE CARE AND FEEDING OF A PRIVATE PRACTICE

Most of us have little difficulty handling the "care and feeding" of our automobiles. Every four or five thousand miles we take the car in to have it oiled, lubed and tuned. When the fuel gauge dips to a certain level, to avoid a long walk, we pull in at a local filling station.

In a similar manner we take pretty good care of the driver. Before getting behind the wheel, we are careful to put on eyeglasses, if we must. We get plenty of rest so that we stay awake at the wheel. And, of course, we're careful to keep the driver sober at all times! For many their relationship with their car is perhaps the healthiest of all their relationships.

What about our relationship with the practice? After a practice has begun to grow there are certain care and maintenance procedures that need to be observed as one does with his own car. Like the driver, what kind of special attention does the therapist require to safely and efficiently manage the practice?

Let's consider this chapter a kind of "Owner's Maintenance Manual." The suggestions offered here are intended to keep the practice and the practitioner healthy, to make a good practice better, and in so doing provide the best care to a needy community. You've got the nuts and bolts for a successful private psychotherapy practice. Now here are the adjustments and the oil to keep it running smoothly.

The 100% Responsibility Rule

A group of psychologists got together over coffee at a local V.A. Hospital where they were all employed. The subject of private practice came up. Several of those present had attempted independent practices but had failed. One therapist cited the lack of community acceptance as the reason for the failure. Another pointed to the "glut" of therapists in the city. A third believed that those patients who did come to his new practice were "not sufficiently motivated for treatment" and were poor referrals.

Notice that there was no shortage of justifications or rationalizations for practice demise. Note also that all the explanations were centered on *externals;* i.e., factors outside the control of the therapists themselves. If our practice is in trouble and we continue to focus our attention on the community, the patients' lack of readiness, or on the competition, we are helpless to resolve the difficulty—because *we can't change externals!*

Someone has said that when we point a finger at someone else we have three fingers pointing back at us! When Edison conducted his experiments in electricity in search of the electric light bulb he never permitted himself the luxury of blaming his many failures on the inadequacy of electricity. No. He attributed the difficulty to *himself,* corrected *his own* errors, and today I have sufficient light to type this manuscript for you.

In order to get a handle on any potential problems in our own practice we use what we call *The 100% Responsibility Rule.* Basically this principle states that any hindrance to practice growth or patient recovery rests squarely on the therapist himself. We look in the mirror and discern how the one looking back at us has allowed whatever condition to develop, and what he must do about it to correct it. The shift is from an external to an *internal* locus of control.

The first step in this procedure is to get our defenses down, throw out all the "excuses" and alibis (and that's no small trick!), and then to ask ourselves the following searching questions:

"Exactly and specifically HOW am I contributing to this problem?"

"What have I done to bring this situation about?"

"WHAT haven't I done to foresee or prevent this difficulty?" The answers to these introspections provide the raw material with which to rebuild the practice and protect its future. Then this data is used to formulate answers to the following probing questions:

"What can I do NOW to correct this situation?"

"What have I learned from these problems and mistakes to use for future practice growth?"

"Where can I turn for counsel, professional advice, business know-how or outside assistance to help me avoid future problems?"

In self-employment we must accept full responsibility for the success or failure of the enterprise. If we keep the emphasis on the guy in the mirror we find ourselves in a powerful position to bring about rapid recovery. No, the 100% Responsibility Rule is never comfortable — accountability never is — but it gets results!

Why not pause here for a few moments and consider. To succeed in a professional practice, are you willing to shoulder *one hundred percent* of the burden? Think about it . . .

The Weekly Review

The 100% Responsibility Rule is essentially an attitude in which the therapist holds himself clearly accountable for practice development. In order for this attitude to become translated into constructive action there needs to be some systematic approach to assessing his performance (or lack of it). The *Weekly Review* offers such an approach.

Basically, the *Weekly Review* calls for the therapist to set aside a block of time each week to put the practice, and himself, under the microscope of accountability. Each week the therapist designates one or two hours during that week for practice review. He then enters this time in the appointment book as he would any paying patient. And he uses that time block for *nothing but practice review*. The time he gives to practice review may not show up on the books as readily as session fees do, but the reward down the line is far greater than the hourly fee could hope to be!

During the *Weekly Review* the therapist scrutinizes and weighs every phase of his practice, always with an eye toward growth and improvement, and always with a positive, open-minded, and enthusiastic attitude. Goals are set and objectives defined. Weaknesses are identified before they turn into wreckage. And the results of practice building efforts are assessed and re-assessed.

Figure 8 gives you a possible framework around which to design a comprehensive *Weekly Review*. At first glance it may seem to you more work than it's worth. But count the cost! Count the cost of a professional practice that slowly withers on the vine due to neglect; versus the booming practice that yields an abundant harvest!

I remember my first attempts at growing tomatoes. During that first season I neglected the dusting, weeding, tying and pruning. The harvest was puny, to say the least. But last year I pruned and pinched and weeded and dusted and really babied all nine plants. And we had tomatoes coming out of our ears!

FIGURE 8. **WEEKLY REVIEW FORMAT**

I. Goal Assessment.
   A. Review the goals from last week. Which ones were met?
   B. Which goals are still unmet? Why? How can I satisfy them this week?
   C. Goals for next week: Phone calls, letters, presentations.

II. Evaluation of Practice Growth.
   A. How many new referrals this week? Referred by whom? How did referral source learn of me? Send letters of acknowledgement. Is feedback to referral source in order?
   B. How many new referrals were via word of mouth by patients? Have I thanked patient? How many from professionals? Time to take them out to lunch as appreciation?
   C. How did I handle telephone screening interviews? Were they too lengthy? How could I improve phone screening?
   D. (Examine appointment book) What did *I* do or not do to contribute to each no-show? Cancellation? Premature (AMA) termination? How did *my own* attitude, style, manner, techniques, and personality affect these factors? What did *I* do (not do) in those sessions that were great successes? In those that were great failures? What can I do this week to improve each situation? Letters to the patients? Phone calls to patients? Prescribed termination? (see pp. 160-162).
   E. Caseload Review (spend time reviewing progress notes for each patient). What *more* can I do to accelerate rapid and permanent change? Do I need consultation on any particular case? Time to re-assess Rx objectives for any particular patient? Cases that should be terminated? Have significant others been brought in as part of pt's Rx? Are charts up to date? If not, I will now set aside from _____ to _____ this coming week for charting (enter time). Contacted all professionals involved with patient to give feedback and courtesy?— schedule each contact now.
   F. Contacts. What opportunities did I use (not use) last week to ethically inform others of my practice? How could I improve this outreach? Log each contact. Is follow-up needed in personal meeting? Phone call? Letter? In each contact was my attitude warm, friendly and professional?
   G. Time spent with colleagues. Sufficient? Schedule lunch with _____ for next week.
   H. Specify and schedule *3* new contacts for practice promotion for next week (see Handbook for ideas).
   I. Where can I offer my services for presentations? Schedule three calls next week.
   J. How much time donated to charity or low income pts last week? How can I increase this next week?
   K. How's my professional growth coming along? Spent time in journal review? Set aside _____ hrs next week. Any workshops, meetings or conventions coming up? Apply this week to _____. Time to enroll for continuing education? Time to consider my own therapy?
   L. Administrative details up to date? Ledger? Checkbook? Charting? Bills paid? Filing? Insurance? Billing? Office supplies?
   M. Have I spent *quality time* with and given my *best* to my family? How can I improve it this week? List 3 special, loving things I will do for spouse this week _____.
      For the children _____.
      For parents _____.
   N. Creative Thinking Time. Set aside one or two hours this week to plan, brain-storm, review Handbook to stimulate practice development.

Don't let neglect slowly choke off your practice. Examine the format in Figure 8 and adapt it to your own needs. And at the outset, before you simply file this away as "a good idea," get out your appointment book and enter in large red letters, "WEEKLY REVIEW." And make it a habit. The investment will bear much fruit!

Caseload Review

Reviewing each case has obvious implications with respect to therapeutic progress. There is another important benefit that should not be overlooked. Careful review of each individual case can suggest interesting and effective channels by which to expand the practice and offer service to a larger parameter in the community. After therapist notes treatment goals and progress notes in the chart, the following questions are asked:

"Would patient's progress be aided by contacting any members of his family (with patient's consent)?"

"Would it profit patient for me to see, write to, or call any of his friends, colleagues, employer (with patient's consent)?"

"To assist patient's progress, should I provide feedback, acknowledgement, or make recommendations to other professionals involved in patient's life (with patient's consent)?"

Therapist then jots down names and phone numbers of these individuals somewhere in the chart (the inside front cover is a good spot for this data).

Every patient brings with him or her a unique circle of significant relationships which effect his or her life. The therapist can mobilize family, friends, work associates, and other professionals to work together as a team on behalf of patient. Don't overlook or minimize these relationships in planning for the patient and for the practice.

Figure 9 (p. 156) illustrates some of the important relationships that you might watch for in caseload review.

Creative Thinking Time

For many of us the last time we engaged in the business of creative thinking dates back to the thesis or dissertation! Every now and then we stumble happily onto a new "twist" in clinical technique, but this is purely accidental. When we are engaged in self-employment we cannot afford to allow our creative faculties to lie dormant or to stagnate. If the press (or threat) of the thesis or

FIGURE 9. CASE REVIEW OF PATIENT'S SIGNIFICANT OTHERS

THE PATIENT

FAMILY & PEERS	OTHER PROFESSIONALS	PROBLEM RELATIONSHIPS
____spouse	____physicians	____"worst enemies"
____children	____ex-therapists	____problem relatives
____parents	____hospitals	____boss, supervisor
____close friends	____social workers	____ex-spouse
____old friends	____probation officers	
____colleagues	____attorneys	
____boss,	____clergymen	
supervisors	____teachers	

dissertation successfully stirred up our imagination, then the dream or vision of a thriving professional practice of our own should kindle a fire under our ingenuity!

If it's been ages since you've exercised any original thinking you might ask: How can I begin to generate original ideas to build the practice? Try this. Set aside a specified time period each week, say, one hour each Monday afternoon. One hour for nothing except CREATIVE THINKING. Brain-storming. Fantasizing on "wild" and crazy ideas. Let your mind run where it will. Think on new ways to treat your patients. Ponder possible new treatment techniques, ideas for research, or improvements in known modalities.

Let brand new ideas float to the conscious mind with regard to ways to promote the practice itself. You might take some of the methods suggested in this Handbook and modify them, combine them with one another, or simply use them to generate unique methods of your own design.

The human mind is a wonderfully amazing thing! Three pounds of gray matter than can produce one thought that can change your life! And it only takes one single idea, followed up with positive, persistent action to make a successful practice a reality—practically overnight. Spend one tenth of the energy you put out during your graduate school days invested in creative thinking time and you will soon need a waiting list or associate therapists to handle the demand for your services! Why not begin *NOW!*

Quality Time With Your Family

One vital area in the therapist's sphere of activities that has been largely ignored is his relationship with his own family. It is my personal feeling that if the therapist has continuing problems in his own home he is of little therapeutic value at the office.

Many therapists make the mistake, as do many executives in industry, of becoming married to their practices. Yes, anyone in self-employment pays a "price" for "sailing his own seas." At the same time he must keep certain priorities in sight. In the business of psychotherapy we see the unpleasantness of human suffering magnified. Every day we hear tales of woe of everything from attempted suicide by ingesting Drano, to the heartbreak of the child covered with cigarette burns in the hands of a psychotic mom or dad.

If the therapist in private practice isn't vigilant about time management he will find himself with a busy office and a home filled with strife. We need time at home playing with the kids on the floor. We must have alone-time with our spouse to laugh and joke around and just unwind. Our family NEEDS US. Therapy really begins at home—nurturing and loving and pitching in to help our loved ones.

Let me share with you one "rule of thumb" that undergirds our own practice. Here it is: MY FAMILY FIRST—EVERYTHING AND EVERYONE ELSE, GET IN LINE! May this bit of wisdom find its way into your own life and practice!

Your Own Supervision

How can you KNOW whether you need either ongoing or periodic outside supervision of your work in private practice? Here are some very reliable guidelines by which to assess the need personally. Ask yourself the following questions. Honestly answer each item during your next Weekly Review, and make it a practice to face these questions periodically throughout the year. Questions:

(1) In my practice, many patients only continue in therapy for a a few sessions, and then drop out. YES ☐ NO ☐
(2) Although my patients stay in treatment, most do not seem to make steady progress or reach set goals. YES ☐ NO ☐

(3) I get very few word-of-mouth referrals from present or past patients in my practice. YES ☐ NO ☐

(4) After the initial phone screening many patients fail to show for their first scheduled session.   YES ☐   NO ☐

(5) The number of patients who call me between sessions and are clinging or overly dependent are increasing. YES ☐ NO ☐

(6) Suicidal threats and attempts, as well as crisis calls are numerous among my patients.   YES ☐   NO ☐

(7) In my practice I get very few referrals from other professionals. YES ☐   NO ☐

(8) I get few referrals from community groups. YES ☐ NO ☐

(9) Collecting patient fees is becoming a problem. YES ☐ NO ☐

(10) Time spent at the office is beginning to interfere with my family relationships.   YES ☐   NO ☐

If you checked "YES" to any of the above items, now, NOW is the time to arrange for outside help. Enlist an experienced clinician to supervise your clinical work, and perhaps a competent therapist to help you examine yourself. WE ARE *ALL* SUSCEPTIBLE TO IMPROVEMENT.

Keeping Yourself Up To Date

It's tempting to get complacent once we receive the degree, the professional license and then the business license, to close the door on the classroom forever. But the field of counseling and psychotherapy is so young and growing so fast that we can't afford the luxury of academic retirement.

Regularly attending seminars, workshops, conventions and training programs keeps the private clinician fresh and his clinical skills sharp.

The American Psychological Association in its *Ethical Standards of Psychologists* calls this our professional responsibility:

"The psychologist, committed to increasing man's understanding of man, places high value on objectivity and integrity, and maintains the highest standards in the services he offers . . .

"As a practitioner, the psychologist knows that he bears a heavy SOCIAL RESPONSIBILITY BECAUSE HIS WORK MAY TOUCH INTIMATELY THE LIVES OF OTHERS." (See Chapt. 3, p. 35).

R And R (Reading and Research)

In private practice we do not typically have the benefit of in-service training. So keeping up with developments in the field is a must. We have to discipline ourselves in this regard. Designating time each week for journal reading or library work is a MUST. You might even consider asking the local VA Hospital if you might drop in for their in-service training from time to time.

We have a responsibility to other professionals as much as to our own patients. When we discover new and innovative methods that consistently bring about therapeutic gain, we are bound to share this information with colleagues. If in-depth research is not your idea of "fun," remember that many journals these days are publishing "Short Reports" of work in progress—methods that are getting results but are not necessarily set in a formal research-paper format. And as you take the time and make the time to prepare such reports, remember: Published reports is an excellent means by which to become known among colleagues. Your appointment book may reflect one of your papers!

Lunch With Colleagues

Another fruitful way to keep up with what's happening is getting together with other therapists. Meeting over lunch, coffee, golf or dinner gives you an opportunity to socialize and at the same time get some informal supervision. Useful strategies, problem cases, and "what's new in the literature" is grist for the mill.

Some private therapists report feelings of loneliness after they enter private practice on a full time basis. Weekly or monthly get-togethers may be just the thing to solve this problem.

I hesitate to mention this, but here goes. Picking up the tab is a good way to informally pay an experienced therapist for supervision of your work! It's tax deductible, you know!

Where To Get Business Consultation & Know-How

Your tax dollars support many agencies that are readily available to you for consultation and assistance in your own practice. Expertise and know-how is at your disposal from such groups as local alcoholism and drug clinics, legal aid agencies, social welfare and child protective agencies, probation and parole departments, police agencies, hospital staffs and rehabilitation agencies. When you have questions about an area within their expertise, you will find these professionals more than eager to help out. Helping you represents a welcome break from their "institutional rut"—and there may be no cost to you whatever.

And do you know where you can find the greatest concentration of talent, know-how, and underpaid brains anywhere? Answer: At your local college or university, of course! Expert advice on legal matters, marketing, practice promotion and public relations, accounting and bookkeeping, tax assistance, research and statistical work, computer access, typing services and on and on—all of this is housed in one place, ready for your knock on the door.

And don't overlook the invaluable help available to you from the head librarian at the local university library. We have found them of great help in using visual aids, audio taping and tape duplication, using space in library cubicles for research projects, obtaining art and graphic assistance, and making special arrangements for you to borrow items restricted or on special hold. GET TO KNOW YOUR FRIENDLY UNIVERSITY LIBRARIAN!

Finally, for matters strictly related to the business end of things, get to know *SCORE. SCORE,* Service Core of Retired Executives, is a group of high level retired businessmen formed by the Small Business Administration. They will provide expert know-how at NO COST TO YOU. Consider SCORE's help with problems such as practice PR, marketing, accounting systems, or perhaps efficiency planning. You have, at your request and at no cost, a wealth of experience and practical how-to's in all those years of business experience among the *SCORE* staff. Take advantage of those "old timers" and give them an opportunity to feel productive in helping you.

The Prescribed Premature Termination

Many therapists in private practice report a rather high rate of premature terminations among their patients. Before therapeutic goals can be reached, the patient fails to return, often without any notification to the therapist.

Causes for this phenomenon are as numerous as the personality types that they represent. And the reasons for such unfortunate interruption in treatment is probably shared equally between patient and therapist.

Can the therapist do anything to reduce this problem? The answer is yes. In those cases in which it becomes obvious that motivation is waning, we have found good success in actually *prescribing premature termination!* When we note in caseload review that no-shows, cancellations, late-arrivals, or lack of progress becomes a common pattern, then we take action. Before the patient reaches the point of avoiding, escaping or resisting treatment by dropping out, we will do it for him. When the patient terminates therapy without discussing this decision with therapist, he or she is simply adding another "failure experience" to his life. By anticipating his avoidance and encouraging it, we help transform a disappointment into another positive step toward his growth.

In the early stages the therapist may say something like this to redefine a potential failure into something therapeutic:

"In our work together we have been dealing with some very important issues in your life. Old memories, new experiences, changes in important relationships, and new challenges and opportunities for you personally begin to come to the surface in your work with me in therapy. Many people find that after a time they need a short break in their therapy. They even feel like dropping out of therapy. And that's understandable because you are dealing with such important changes in your life.

"You may get the same kind of feelings from time to time yourself. And that's perfectly all right. If at any time you feel like stopping our work together for a while, fine, do so. Let me know how you feel and we will arrange a "vacation." Take a breather. Step back for a while and take a look at what we have accomplished; try out some of your new insights. Then come back into therapy only when *you* are ready to finish the work you began. Remember, this is *your* therapy.

"Perhaps it would be a good time for you to take a break . . . what do you think?"

Can you see the benefit of this approach for the patient who feels temporarily overwhelmed or threatened? The guilt due to his failure to discuss termination is neutralized. His decision to drop out is verbalized and positively defined as "OK" and becomes part of the treatment process. Termination becomes a "vacation" rather than another "I've messed up another relationship" experience. And best of all, the door is left wide open and accessible for his return to you when he is ready.

This method is also most effective in injecting new life into the treatment process. Patients will be encouraged to take a break when it becomes obvious that they are "coasting" or dragging their feet in therapy. Or the patient may simply have reached a plateau. A prescribed two week or one month time-out from therapy often brings patient back with a new commitment to change; and progress is accelerated.

The Therapeutic Letter

Because of previous conditioning in their relationships with other professionals, most patients expect their relationship with therapist to begin and end at the consultation room. However, when they receive a personal, caring and sincere expression of the therapist's concern for them in the mail, the impact is remarkable!

Most patients, after all, are patients because they suffer a lack of love or genuine attention in their little world. When the therapist takes the time to drop the patient a personal note of encouragement, hope, and positive regard, the therapeutic gain is often dramatic. Dropping a line or two to a patient is something I do not particularly enjoy doing—since my letter writing track record is terrible even within my own family! But I schedule time for the activity because of the tremendous results that ensue. It has been my own experience that intermittent notes to patients rapidly builds a therapeutic relationship, increases trust, deepens patient commitment to treatment, motivates patient to follow through on assigned homework, and often prevents premature termination.

For example, when Bob failed to keep a scheduled session, as discussed above, a short note was sent to him defining his decision as understandable and the best one at that time (see Figure 10).

During his Weekly Review time a therapist noted that a patient called for an appointment, was given complete screening and scheduled for their first session, but failed to show. Figure 11

FIGURE 10. PREMATURE TERMINATION LETTER

(LETTERHEAD)

20 November 1981

Dear Bob:

During our usual appointment time last week I took the opportunity to look over your chart and notes from our work together. I wanted to drop you this note to share with you some of my thoughts about your progress.

Since the first time you began therapy I notice that you have made some significant changes. They have not been easy, I know, but they will form the foundation for future strength and growth in your life.

It's also apparent that some of the matters that we've been dealing with lately are somewhat difficult to understand and deal with. That is common in therapy. You are at a most important phase in your progress now.

Your decision to take a breather from therapy for a while I think is a good one. Take some time before you return to resume your therapy to put into practice the things we have worked on together. Take a vacation from therapy for a while and when you begin anew, you'll be ready to complete therapy with more energy and with renewed ability.

Until that time, I am always available to you if I can be of assistance in any way at all.

Best personal regards,

FIGURE 11. INITIAL-NO-SHOW LETTER

(LETTERHEAD)

7 June 1981

Dear Mrs. Schwartz:

Just a short note to thank you for calling regarding our services and how they might be of benefit to you.

Beginning the important work in therapy is often a difficult decision. And even once that decision is made, it can be somewhat awkward or uncomfortable to come in for that first session. I know. Many people find the first session unsettling until they actually get involved in the situation. Then things get easier.

Now that you've made the important decision to work out some of the areas of concern in your life, do pursue therapy when you are ready. It does not have to be with our clinic, of course. But it is a good idea to begin as soon as possible with someone who is skilled to help you work toward a more rewarding life.

Before coming to your first session, it might help you to jot down notes in outline form to help you organize your thoughts. This helps use time well and it can help relax you a bit also.

If there is any way in which we can be of service to you, please feel free to call any time.

Cordially yours,

illustrates a note of encouragement to this prospective patient. Due to the concern expressed by therapist, patient called to re-schedule another appointment—and followed through!

During periods of Weekly Review therapist may also note certain patients who have not been consistent in folloiwng through with assigned homework as part of therapy. A short note of positive encouragement might help. And whenever you run across a magazine or newspaper article, cartoon, poem or what-have-you that triggers a certain patient in your mind, drop it in the mail to the patient. Its message, plus the covert message that YOU CARE! will produce dramatic therapeutic effects.

Letters of "best regards" or "just thinking of you" for no particular reason to former patients, some that you have perhaps not seen for years, is a great idea. Somehow they seem to reach the person in a time of need and bring renewed hope.

And don't overlook letters or questionnaires to patient's spouses and family members. It's a good way to get significant others involved on patient's behalf (see pp. 97-99).

Unless you love to correspond, we recommend that you enter a specified time in your appointment book, say, Wednesday, 12:30 to 1 p.m., "TREATMENT LETTERS." Then force yourself to get out at least one a week. Keep the letters as personal, warm and friendly, and as unlike form letters as possible.

If you make Therapeutic Letters a part of your practice protocol, you will see a two-fold result. First, you will realize some unusual gains in both the therapeutic relationship with your patients, and in their overall treatment progress. And secondly, because of "going the extra mile" for your patients, because you choose to do "more than just enough" for them, you may soon find yourself in a higher income bracket!

In summary, if I had to isolate one variable which would insure the success of your practice, and that would enrich your own life personally, I think it could be summed up in this epitaph. Listen closely:

"What I spent, I lost;
What I possessed is left to others;
What I freely gave away remains with me."

CHAPTER ELEVEN

HOW TO FILL YOUR APPOINTMENT BOOK
CASE STUDIES SHOWING HOW THE BUSIEST THERAPISTS ATTRACT NEW PATIENTS AND BUILD GROWING CLIENTELES

CHAPTER 11
HOW TO FILL YOUR APPOINTMENT BOOK
CASE STUDIES SHOWING HOW THE BUSIEST
THERAPISTS ATTRACT NEW PATIENTS
AND BUILD GROWING CLIENTELES

Before the ink was dry on the first printing of *Private Practice Handbook* we had accumulated a file of new and innovative methods that therapists around the country were using to get some marvelous results in building their practices. These ideas and approaches were not all new—some were simply a combination of other procedures already reported in the first edition, or they were an offshoot of promotion methods used by other professionals in their own practice development work.

Many of these successful and busy therapists have learned an important truth in the promotion of their practice:

"What works; what gets results; what attracts new clients or patients in one professional sphere may work in building my own practice."

In this chapter we will present for you a collection of case studies of mental health professionals who have learned to fill their appointment books by finding novel, "Rube Goldberg" methods to get their practice name maximum exposure in their communities. Getting exposure for your practice involves practice promotion, publicity, PR or public relations, and advertising.

The Name Of The Game Is Practice Promotion

Practice PR (public relations) is a subject about as welcome as a pork chop at a bar mitzvah with most clinicians. There seems to be a quasi-Hippocratic oath among many therapists that "Thou shalt not promote thine own work." An attitude develops in some professionals, that "If I'm this good, have all these degrees and licenses, and this swanky office—how can I help but make it big; they'll beat a path to my door." Oh, would that it were so easy!

The fact is, however, if you don't systematically work at telling them how good, degreed, licensed and swank you are, the only one beating a path to your door will be the mailman, bringing with him handfuls of bills, due and payable.

Let's take a look at a perfect example of good PR and promotions in action. I think you'll enjoy it. It appeared in the December, 1981 edition of *Reader's Digest:*

"One departure check-in area of the Phoenix airport is kept pleasantly quiet, and even the Salvation Army volunteer found that her familiar bells weren't allowed. As a result, she attracted little attention during her first day's duty. The next day, her business was brisk as she waved two signs in the air. One read DING, the other DONG."

Now that's good promotion; good PR! That's the way to get attention. And that's the way to fill her pot!

That's also the way to get attention and fill your own appointment book (and your own pot!) as well.

She could have gone home that night and said, "I better give up on this location—nobody's giving anything here. Better try another location tomorrow." Or, like some determined, but not-yet-successful private practices, she could have just stood there day after day with a big smile on her face, content with only a few tokens of man's compassion at the bottom of her empty pot. But instead, what did she do to promote a "brisk business"?

We're all used to the *sound* of the DING, DONG. But how often have you seen two signs held up calling out in bold letters, *DING, DONG*? What did she do to get attention and fill the pot? She made her job, her particular business a little bit different. She gave it a "twist." She built curiosity value into her work. In short, she used promotion, publicity and PR to make her work successful.

And if your practice is to do the same thing, you must know how to do what she did. So let's examine in detail how some of the most creative—and busy—professionals build booming clienteles and how they use the *"DING-DONG"* method in doing so.

As you read, keep your eyes open, (pencil in hand), for possible modifications or twists that *you* might implement in your own practice, as well as using their methods outright.

Advertising A Seminar Series—The Spin-Off Principle

We've been talking so far about promotions, publicity and PR. Now advertising *per se* does not fall within these categories. The former involve getting practice exposure for *free**, while advertising costs, and costs plenty! Both approaches are used every day by successful clinicians to get the attention of those who need their services, and both are potent practice builders, when used within definite ethical boundaries. Here's how one enterprising Pastoral Counselor, Marriage Therapist got 140,000 neighbors to learn about his forthcoming seminar series:

On the left-hand page of a large metropolitan newspaper appears a 7" X 3½" display ad. Over at the right we see a drawing of a father with his little boy sitting on his shoulders with the number "19" on his shirt, and a look of pure joy on the little guy's face. At the top of the ad, in striking bold, half-inch letters we read the headline:

BECOME A BETTER PARENT!

Alongside the dad and his boy, we see the rest of the ad and learn how we can become a better parent—

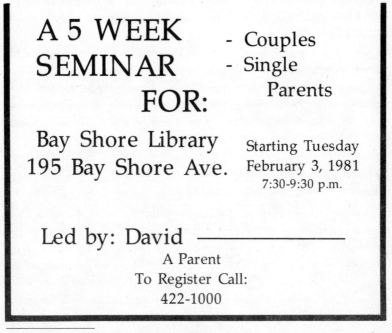

*If you're interested in a detailed course in the "How To's" of getting free publicity for your practice, write to Duncliff's for free information.

This ad reached a potential audience of 140,000 people. The cost of the ad was $296. Was it worth the investment for this therapist? Let's see: As a result of this ad the therapist had a well attended seminar in the library for five weeks running. He charged *nothing* to those attending. How was it successful? As a result of this seminar he started a couples group at his office for which he charged the standard rate, and received three, one-to-one, paying patients besides! Although this ad could stand much improvement as far as good ad construction goes, still, it did the job nicely. This investment showed a substantial profit within two weeks!

Here's a point to remember when thinking about an advertising campaign for your work. First of all, review your ethical guidelines as they pertain to your specialty. Then if advertising is permitted, make sure you use some headline and topic matter that will: a) get attention fast, b) hold the interest of a wide group of people, c) has some "news" value, and d) is affordable, or preferably free to the reader, as in the above case, to screen *in* as many people as possible who need your help. Try to make your topic or program specific and not general. A "How To" or "You Can Overcome..." or "New Ways to Handle..." title for your ad and your seminar or talk will usually bring in many inquiries.*

Speaking of inquiries: It is always best to give a phone number for more information. This will help overcome the natural reluctance of the reader, and will give you some idea of how many to plan for. If the caller is not interested in your seminar, he or she may be interested in your other work. Your secretary or whomever answers your phone should be ready to give out this information.

Lecture Series Announcements
Brings a "Sick" Enterprise Back To Life

A private psychiatric hospital in Southern California looked as if it was going the way of the Titanic, primarily because of poor management and terrible publicity. When it was taken over by a group of sharp professionals, one of the first things that they did was to hire a good PR firm. After analyzing why the Titanic went (or almost went) down, it was recommended that the hospital had to get the good favor of the professional community. Such favor had long since been lost.

*If you need help in preparing effective advertising for your work, Duncliff's offers such consultation by mail. You can write for more details.

How to court the local professional mental health community? It was decided to institute a series of Lectures, bringing in some of the most famous and honored clinicians in the country. A month or so before each Lecture, an announcement was sent out to every mental health professional within a 200 mile radius.

The announcement was printed on the finest ivory parchment enclosed in an envelope of the same quality paper. Each was addressed individually (no mailing labels used) and sent first class mail.

Inside a handsome border this is what you find—

You Are Invited To Attend A Free. . . .
LECTURE SERIES
Lecture 3

William ————, Ph.D.

"LETTING GO OF LOVE AND OTHER MYTHS'"
Dr. ———— is the author of ————
He is also in private practice.

January 13, 1982
7:30 p.m.
Marshall High School - Auditorium
9877 East High Boulevard

Sponsored By

—————— HOSPITAL
6000 Lakewood Boulevard
Lakewood, California 90000
For more information, please call (213) 634-9000

After attending a series of FREE lectures of this sort, sitting under some of the finest minds in the field, and of course, hearing periodically about the many new programs and policies at this hospital, and being offered staff membership and privileges. . . .what do you suppose was the result? You're absolutely right—when these local professionals needed in-hospital care for their own patients, where do you suppose they sent them? Right again!

Now you may not be interested in running a hospital at this point. So how could this same tactic be used by a small group of professionals in private practice? Exactly the same way as the hospital used it. Arrange with a well-known authority in the mental health field to speak on a given evening. Arrange to rent a local auditorium for that night. Using the Direct Mail Announcement* send a similar announcement to every appropriate professional within driving distance, giving a phone number for further information. During the evening's presentation, include some interesting presentation that highlights your own practice and its special techniques, programs, seminars, etc.

Referrals flow into a practice primarily because of the exposure the practice receives. No need to follow up your lecture series with calls or letters. Now they know you exist; that's enough.

Anatomy of a News Release:
The Cheapest & Most Effective Way to Get Free Publicity

The unwritten law in every newspaper in this country is this: Every day they have to fill space in their paper with "newsy" information. Their staff writers and their ad salesmen can fill just so much space. Therefore, when they receive something of interest to the public in the form of a "News Release" they are quite pleased. "Ah, that's just right for that dead space on page nine in the "Neighborhood News" Section, let's run it. . ."

So when you have something that's of interest to Mr. and Mrs. Citizen, get out a News Release to every paper in your area. It doesn't matter if one or all of them run it. And the beauty of this tool is that IT'S FREE!

Here's an actual News Release used by another hospital to get local professionals involved in their new mental health programs and units. You'll note how brief and to the point it is. Nothing fancy. Just facts— What, When, Where, How Much, Who. . . . That's it. You can use this sample of an actual News Release to model your own in order to get some great exposure for your work. Here it is:

---

*Direct Mail and other media promotion ideas are detailed for you in Duncliff's "How To Build A Practice Clientele Using Key Referral Sources—A Sourcebook." See pp. 234-237.

NEWS RELEASE * * * NEWS RELEASE * * * NEWS RELEASE

For information
John Dokes, Director
(213) 332-8924

"Innovative Approaches to Managing Pain" will be the topic at the Wed., Feb. 3, monthly community education series at ——— Hospital in San Diego. The seminar will begin at 8:30 a.m. with a free continental breakfast in the hospital's main dining area.

Joseph C. ————, Ph.D., assistant professor of psychology, Yale University Center for Behavioral Medicine, and director of the Yale Psychological Training and Research Institute, will be the scheduled speaker at the seminar.

Dr. ———— has written numerous articles and papers on stress, anxiety and pain and has lectured extensively on these subjects.

The seminar is open to all health professionals and to the general public. For more information or reservations, call the ——— Hospital Community Services office at: (714) 332-8924.

#   #   #

This hospital sent this News Release to every local paper, including the "throw aways." Notice that the seminar is open to the general public. The hospital's primary aim was the health care professionals, right? But becoming known to the laymen can also bring in some good business. But keep this in mind when doing seminars and using the News Release to promote them: If you include in your News Release the fact that Mr. & Mrs. Citizen are also invited, you're much more likely to get this information printed for you. If it's a highly esoteric, "closed" meeting, they may publish it only in their round file! So if you can, open the doors wide to as many folks as possible.

Two Professionals Join Forces And Prosper

A recent article in the *Los Angeles Times* began this way:

"It was all over for Bill and Arvilla Simsic. Their marriage of 21 years that had produced three children had hit the skids. . .So since they planned to dissolve their union, they chose a method which they considered a more agreeable way to disagree. They chose divorce mediation—A system whereby a trained professional with a background in law or counseling acts as a neutral mediator and assists the couple in contractually settling the issues of their divorce."

L.A. Times: January 7, 1982

This fascinating article goes on to tell the heartbreaking story of this split family, and more importantly for our purposes, we are told how two professionals united their separate skills and are now flooded with referrals.

Essentially what happened is this. A California attorney and a Marriage Therapist got together to form a Mediation Service. Rather than each party in a divorce getting his or her own lawyer and fighting it out, costing thousands of dollars and costing the kids a lot of grief as well, the couple agrees to use the same attorney and his therapist associate to work out their parting on a friendly basis—saving the horendous cost of the legal battle in the courts, and saving years of bitter resentments.

The couple sees the attorney and the therapist on separate occasions and works out the terms of the divorce in peace. In addition to avoiding the battle in the courts, the couple can save (according to the professionals) from $1,000 to $98,000 using the mediation approach.

Looking at the above from the perspective of the therapist, we see some interesting things. Rather than the therapist getting locked in to his traditional role of the counselor, trying with all his wits to prevent the divorce, he uses those skills to help the couple adjust to their divorce. He also offers his talents of peacemaker and communications expert to the attorney, whose expertise lies in the legal machinery. They can help the unhappy couple legally, emotionally, and financially. And in the process, each professional involved has to give up his Wednesday golf date and those 3-hour lunches, because he's so busy he can't afford to take the time off! Not bad!

How's the Mediation Business faring in your area? Know any crack attorneys that might be interested in joining forces with a crack mental health professional that you just might happen to know? And suppose there is a Mediation Service already operating at present? Even in the professional world. . . .*competition;* that's what keeps America so great, isn't it?

How To Use "Publicity Leverage"
To Build Your Practice

Let's pause for a few moments and look at the flip side of what we've been talking about here. In the three cases we have just discussed a professional therapist has, by hook or by crook or by a good PR firm, gotten some great exposure (promotion) for his practice, right? Let's also suppose that you are not so inclined to get such publicity, but you would like to have some strategy by which you could benefit from *their* fame. Remember, because of this kind of publicity, they are likely to find themselves buried under a torrent of interest in their work. They will undoubtedly get calls and inquiries from many people whom they cannot serve now, or who are not appropriate for their work. Shouldn't they have *someone* standing ready to take those referrals? Now you see the picture. To illustrate, let's apply the method. . . .

In the case of the "Become a Better Parent" clinician: How could you let him know about your work? You could pick up the phone and ask him to refer anyone he cannot help to you. But most professionals don't have the crust or the thick skin to do that kind of thing. So here's a better approach—that works. Why not pick up the phone and call the number in the ad. Get in touch with the professional himself and say something like this,

> "Hi David, this is Dr. ————. I saw your notice in today's paper. . .it really sounds like an interesting group! *(Pause)* I wonder if you might have a few minutes to tell me a bit about the plans for the group—you see, I am a *(your specialty)* and I may be able to refer some of my patients to your group. What kind of couples are you looking for. . .?"

The group indeed could benefit one of your own patients. And if not, no harm done, he now knows *you* exist, doesn't he? After he gives you the information about his group, ask if he has any literature, any brochures or syllabus for the program that you might have to hand out to those who are interested, or to put in your waiting room. He'll then send them to your office address. Then when you receive them, you quickly shoot him back a letter of appreciation—which also contains your business card! In the letter you may also want to mention getting together over lunch in a few weeks to share ideas, etc., etc.

Now here's someone who has all the work he can handle as a result of a good advertising campaign. Before today he never heard of you or your work, did he? But within a week's time, he not only knows about you, he's taken the time to send you some materials, knows where your office is, and has received a warm correspondence from you, and may even be planning to go out to a lunch, *on you,* the following week. That's called "publicity leverage."

What about the hospital Lecture Series? You know that they are sponsoring those "Free" lectures for a purpose—to reach you and other professionals so that you will refer any patients who need in-patient care to them. Okay. Why not call that "For more information" number and thank them for the invitation, requesting more details; also asking about upcoming Lectures. Should you have referred one of your patients to another hospital recently, tell the hospital PR person that you regret not knowing about their services. Then, ask them about their services in detail and take notes while they are talking. Ask about staff privileges and membership. After you have created a warm and friendly relationship with this person on the phone, ask if he or she will be at the upcoming lecture. Arrange to meet them there and continue refining the relationship. Then they will doubtless invite you to join the staff and may, and here's the important step, introduce you to the key people there who typically make *out*patient referrals to those in private practice. *Voila!*

And finally, here's how the Mediation Service article was handled successfully by one psychologist. Immediately after reading the article, the therapist made time in his schedule to get out this letter to the attorney himself—

January 8, 1982

WE WERE INTRIGUED BY YOUR
MEDIATION WORK, MR. ————. . .

Until we saw your article we were not aware of your work in ———— County. Great to know that you are nearby, and I can assure you of one thing—we sure can keep you busy!

We are a group of psychologists and marriage therapists here in the North County. Most of our patients are referred to us by the Conciliation Court and from private physicians and attorneys. Our job, of course, is to make an all out effort to put the family that's in trouble back together and head off the divorce, if possible. But as you know, more and more this seems a tough nut to crack.

We are involved all the time in messy and heartbreaking child custody matters and bitter divorce cases. Your work sounds just like what we have been looking for to help those troubled families and couples that cannot seem to begin again together to at least part in peace—and to keep the innocent little ones out of the cross fire.

I would be grateful if you would kindly let us know how we might go about making referrals to your group? Perhaps you have some brochures you could send along that we might have handy here at the office to hand out to our patients who are suitable for this service; and that we might place in our reception area?

And it would be good to meet with you one of these days soon to share ideas—your training in Maryland certainly sounds fascinating! Look forward very much to hearing from you, and I'll give you a call early next week to work out a good time to get together for lunch at your convenience.

And again, many thanks!

Yours, with best regards,

Dr. — — — — — — — —
Director

Before there was even a chance to make the luncheon date the attorney shot back 15 copies of a beautiful brochure along with the following letter. Notice how the informality and warm spirit of the above letter established this relationship so quickly. Here's the reply letter:

LAW OFFICES OF ——————

January 14, 1982

Dear Dr. ————:

First of all, thank you very much for your considerate and encouraging letter of January 8, 1982.

We believe that mediation is a much needed alternative to the traditional "adversary" divorce system.

To make referral to the ———— Family Mediation Service, you merely have your patients or clients telephone the service at 714-————. We will be happy to take it from there.

I would like very much, as you suggest, to meet with you some time soon and share our ideas. Meanwhile, I am enclosing herein several brochures which you may feel free to pass out to anyone requesting one.

Very Truly Yours,

———— ————————

Using publicity leverage you can systematically expand your circle of new friends while getting tremendous exposure for your own practice at the same time. Don't forget to use the lunches as tax deductions! And keep your eye on each day's newspaper—you'll find in almost every issue endless possibilities to get your practice known using publicity leverage.* Or perhaps you might be interested in getting direct publicity and promotion for your own work? If so, you'll enjoy the next section. . . .

How to Get Free Publicity
By Riding the Crest of a Fad

We go into far greater detail on how to get free publicity and promotion for your practice in Duncliff's Promotion and Publicity Manual. But to give you the mechanics of the procedure, let's take a

---

* In the interim, The Mediation Service invited this therapist to join them, receive their training, and become a satellite center. Now that's leverage at its best!

specific example of how one psychologist boosted referrals to his part-time practice by taking advantage of a present day fad. Look at this article that appeared in the *Long Beach* (California) *Press Telegram:* Circulation—140,000 daily. At the very top of the article we see a close-up photo of the posterior portions of a young man and woman, both dressed in tight fitting "designer jeans." Then the headline—

"PROF SAYS DESIGNER LABELS MASK INSECURITY"

A USC psychology professor claims that people who wear designer labels are covering up a feeling of insecurity. Instead of being "with it," they're really "out of it."

Chayton D. ————, who has a clinical practice in Pomona, says people who buy status through their clothes are really saying, "You may not like me, but you'll like what I've bought."

Press Telegram: December 27, 1981

This article goes on and on in this profound vein; we won't bore you with the rest. Suffice it to say that this therapist got a pretty good exposure for his Pomona clinical practice on the coat-tails of the hula hoop of the '80's, designer jeans. And why not? Everyone is interested in this subject today—if they were not, the paper would never had done the story on this professor-clinician.

What was the outcome? Well, you can be sure that those who advertise Jordache, Sergio Valenti, and Calvin Klein on their backsides will not find their way to his office in Pomona, right? But what about the older set who may happen to agree with Dr. So and So? What about all those parents who are worried about their kids' poor self-image already? We have no data at this date, but we would probably be close to the mark if we conclude that our anti-designer colleague is mighty busy these days working on building new self-images and helping many folks find their uniqueness!

Before we showed you this strategy, you might have said, "How in the world could I use designer jeans to build my practice—you've gotta be kidding!" But now you can see for yourself how one very clever colleague of yours rode this fad right into his waiting room. Along with every fad or craze or public whim there is a psychological angle that motivates it. If you will keep your eyes open while watching the nightly news, or reading *Time,* or your local paper, you might be able to find just that angle yourself.

When you find the angle, the certain something intriguing about the news or fad that you can hook into, then what? Two ways to go: First, if you know the public relations and promotions business, you can send out a news release and get a paper to cover your story....or perhaps you can write the story yourself and they'll run it. Next, should you, as most clinicians are, be totally at a loss in the world of public relations, you can hire a good professional PR firm, tell them your special angle, and pay them to make the necessary contacts for you to get the article in front of your community. Be sure, however, to keep your eyes on those ethical standards! Remember, you not only represent yourself and your practice, you represent the entire profession.

If our anti-label friend had paid for an advertisement in the same paper instead of using some good PR promotion savvy, it would have cost him hundreds of dollars; and the people who don't read ads would never have seen it. But almost everyone reads NEWS. So his PR dollar was well spent, wasn't it? Over 100,000 possible readers!

Do you know how the Mayo Clinic was built? What about Menningers, Schick and the Masters and Johnson Institute? *Public Relations and Promotion.* Master those skills yourself, or hire good PR brains—they're the most powerful tool in building your own practice!

How to Compete With the Competition

In the world of professional practice we don't much like talking about "competition." We are supposed to be above such things, more dignified and unconcerned about who gets what referrals. That's fine if we are trying to impress the layman with our pristine image. But when we get down to the *business* of filling that appointment book, paying the office rent and the home mortgage, let's face it—we are competing for referrals just as Ford and General Motors compete with Lincolns and Cadillacs! But, of course, we do it with *finesse*....Case in Point—

On her initial intake interview, the therapist learned that Charlotte had been referred to him by her best friend, who was also a patient of the therapist. In further questioning, it was learned that Charlotte was an airline stewardess and that she had been first referred by her Employee Assistance Manager to a psychiatrist who practiced near the airport.

The course of therapy went very well until Charlotte was transferred to Colorado. During Practice Development Time the week following her termination, the therapist asked himself this question:

"Is there any way that I can get a foot in the door with the United Airlines Employee Assistance Manager now that Charlotte is transferred and not under my care?" What would you do in this case? Can you see any way to get that EAP Manager to use YOU as one of their referral sources?

Here's what our therapist did. First, he sent out this letter to the Employee Assistance Manager—

September 4, 1981

Mrs. —————,
    Employee Assistance Manager
United Airlines
1234 Airport Drive
Los Angeles, California 90000

Re: Charlotte ————

Dear Mrs. ————:

For your records, I'd like to bring you up to date on the progress of Charlotte's therapy with me.

As you know, Charlotte was first referred to Dr. ———— in the Airport Plaza Building. Because this was so inconvenient for her, being too far from her home, she was referred to this clinic for evaluation and counseling.

I saw her myself in individual consultation from 5/3/81 until just last week. She has now been transferred, as you probably know, to the Denver area. Prior to her transfer, Charlotte made especially good progress in her work with me—eliminating absenteeism altogether, and smoothing out the marital problems which she shared with you prior to seeing me, and which led to problems on the job.

I am attempting to assist her now in locating a qualified and skilled therapist in the Denver area. As soon as I have helped her get settled in that relationship, I will give you a call to let you know the details, so that you can bring your records up to date.

I hope that this information will be helpful to you in assisting in her transfer, and, should you have any questions, please do call me at the above number. Until we speak on the phone soon, I am

Yours sincerely,

——— —————, Ph.D.
Director of Clinical Services

Once again, how did the therapist get this new referral source open to using him? He did not ask for the referrals, did he? He offered to *give service;* information, the details on Charlotte's new therapist, to help her bring her records on Charlotte up to date. To get a foot into a door that another therapist or therapists have dominated for years, use this formula. And make this the motto of your practice:

ALWAYS GIVE SERVICE!

Remember the Seed Principle? Give service. And after you give service in a letter, follow it up with a phone call, giving more service. Taking them out to lunch is optional; giving service is an absolute necessity!*

An Inexpensive Way to Make
Yellow Pages Advertising Pay Off:
The Therapist Consortium Referral Service

You'll recall that earlier in this book we recommended that you steer clear of Yellow Pages telephone advertising for your practice because (1) it is extremely costly, and (2) it is typically ineffective in bringing in new referrals to warrant the investment. However, recently some enterprising therapists with good business heads have come up with a way to overcome the financial bite and make the Yellow Pages pay off.

Take a look at two display ads that appear in the 1982 phone book under the heading, "Marriage, Family & Child Counselors."

*Some time later this therapist spotted an interesting article on Employee Assistance Programs in a professional journal. "Thought you might enjoy this" he wrote on the back of his business card—and mailed it to the Manager. Promotion at its best!

INFORMATION & REFERRAL
TO STATE LICENSED MARRIAGE, FAMILY & CHILD COUNSELORS

PSYCHOLOGISTS, PSYCHIATRISTS &
CLINICAL SOCIAL WORKERS
A PROFESSIONAL SERVICE THAT HELPS SELECT THE
TYPE OF THERAPY & THERAPIST BEST SUITED FOR YOU
MOST INSURANCE ACCEPTED

—— —— Psychotherapy Assn.

CALL

A CONSUMER ORIENTED
SERVICE TO ASSURE
INDIVIDUALLY AFFORDABLE
FEES WITH HIGHLY
QUALIFIED THERAPISTS

313-2100

"AN ORGANIZATION
DEDICATED TO HIGH ETHICAL
& PROFESSIONAL STANDARDS"

INFORMATION & REFERRAL

State Licensed Marriage, Family
& Child Counselors
Psychiatrists, Clinical Social Workers,
Clinical Psychologists

**REFERRAL TO THERAPISTS
RECOGNIZED BY MOST
INSURANCE COMPANIES
A NATIONALLY RECOGNIZED
NON-PROFIT SERVICE**
TO ASSURE LOW FEES
DAY OR NIGHT CALL

429-1111

PSYCHOTHERAPY AFFILIATION
332 NORTH ATLANTIC

You say, "But this is just an "Information & Referral' service....how does this benefit the private practitioner, and how could this benefit my practice?" Yes, you're exactly correct; it is an information and referral service. But if you read between the lines, and look behind the outward appearances, you'll see something quite interesting....

Ask yourself this: Who put the display ad in the phone book? Who pays the bill each month to run it? When someone calls, looking for "the type of therapy and therapist best suited" for them, who do you think they are referred to?

Do you see it? Here's how it works. Because the crushing blow of inflation has forced the consumer to become highly cautious as to how he or she spends every dollar, they are also more than ever careful about how they go about selecting someone to help them handle their emotional problems. Seldom any more does someone wander through the Yellow Pages roster and look for a name that suits his fancy—those days are over. The consumer wants some kind of assurance, some hope that the professional he or she selects is "recognized" as competent. So what does Mr. & Mrs. Citizen do? When they look in the phone book they see a service displayed there for them that will help them find the "Best" most "Recognized" and "Licensed" therapist, *"Best for You."* So they feel somehow that they are not picking a "shrink" out of the air. Therefore, the first thing this "Info & Referral" ad does is to build their confidence and overcome their fear of getting "someone who is more messed up than I am"—and that little expression is on the minds of more people today than you might think!

So then, *who* placed the ad to build their confidence and win their trust? It's not a local or national professional association. It's not a consumer protection group. It's a small group of therapists like yourself who get together, in one office or in their separate practices, and decide to provide an information and referral service. Obviously, the information and referrals provided to the callers happily centers around their own group! The cost of the first ad is $129.30 and the second runs $86.20 per month. Split seven, eight or twelve ways the investment is well worth the risk, isn't it?

For this kind of system to work best—best, that is, for the public good—the therapists involved should of course be the most skilled professionally, and further, they should have their separate practices located in different parts of the city or county. In the case of the second ad, this Affiliation consists of fifteen licensed psychologists, psychiatrists, clinical social workers, and MFCC's covering an entire county.

Could any one of these therapists get this kind of exposure for so little investment? Would it be possible to increase public confidence simply using a practice name, or the professional's own name and credentials? It's unlikely.

Take a look in your own phone book. Are there such ads there? Even if there are—and don't forget, we got these two ads off of the same page in the same book—all you have to do is make your ad a bit more attractive and attention-getting than the others there and your phone will be the one that rings.

Using a Non-Profit Corporation
as an Umbrella for Your Practice

If you will take a look at the second display ad in the last section, you will note the little tag line just above the phone number; "Non-Profit Service To Assure Low Fees." You can get along just fine without such a corporate status for your work. And should you like the idea of the therapist consortium referral service, there is no need to go to the trouble to form a non-profit corporation. It is a costly legal matter, especially in the initial formation of the corporation, and requires a lot of paper work to keep the organization ship-shape and legal. Now, on the other hand....

Is it worth the cost and the hassle? Perhaps this will help you decide. Suppose you were looking for the best professional therapist you could find (who walks on water, of course!) and you were looking over these two ads trying to decide which to call. Even though the first is larger—which might cause you to think that you could trust the referral to be more qualified—you would in all psychological likelihood call the second one. Why? Because we are all looking for something "low." Especially fees! Now the non-profit label "to assure low fees" would probably function as the trigger to get the action for this group. It would only take one or two paying patients to easily overcome the cost of and the hassle of the corporation umbrella.

Now forming a non-profit corporation to cover your everyday practice income is not a simple trick. But forming such an organization as the vehicle to operate your group's referral service may not be that difficult to manage. But we will leave you to the good counsel of your attorney and tax consultant on this score.

School Psychologist Builds His Practice
On Dissatisfaction With the Public School System

None of us needs to be reminded these days about the state of the public school's report card with the public—most middle and upper class Americans are not very happy about declining performance, drugs and violence, even at the elementary level. The exodus from public to private schools has grown to such a proportion that laws have recently been passed to block the migration.

Public Law 94-142 is one such ordinance. Essentially, this piece of legislation states that no public school community can be forced to reimburse a private school that a parent selects for his child unless it can be proven that the public school system is unable to provide the special care the student requires. If the child can get the same services from a public school within a reasonable distance from his home, the parent must assume the total cost of the private education, without any tax advantage, if he chooses this route.

One alert school psychologist saw a promising opportunity in this parents-vs-Uncle Sam contest. Representing the public school system, his job was to assemble all the evidence to prove in various fair hearings that the school system could, in fact, give satisfactory service. If he could not prove it, the taxpayers foot the bill for the private school. "Just suppose" he asked himself one payday, "just suppose I use the knowledge I already have, but join the parents in their cause?"

That "Just suppose. . ." turned into a profitable adjunct to his part-time counseling practice. Here's how he did it. He carefully prepared a presentation of his qualifications, the current problem the private schools and parents have in proving that the child cannot get the attention they need at the public schools, and why both needed his services to get an upper hand in the hearings with the school systems. It wasn't difficult for the private school administrators and owners to see that in him they had the answer to their prayers. Thus, as a consultant to the private schools and to the parents they referred to him, he became their expert witness. . . .one who also knew every move the opposition would make.

Aside from the lucrative consultation work, he received many referrals for private counseling with those children (and their parents).

If this idea (or some modification of it) stirs up your curiosity, and you know practically nothing about Public Law 94-142 and related issues that we have discussed here, consider tracking down a school psychologist who has been dreaming about some kind of private practice involvement for years? If you know of no one, you might consider advertising for such a person in the "Position and Career Opportunities" section in the newsletters of professional school psychologist associations and the American Personnel and Guidance Association. As the educational system continues to stagger under bad publicity, this side-line to your practice could keep you quite busy!

Testing Services to Private Schools
Multiplies Psychologist's Caseload

One child psychologist was of the opinion that five and six year old children who are placed into the first grade are being pushed too fast, too soon into an adult mold, and, as a consequence, they suffer both emotional, social and even physical impairment. His thesis was, and is, that children should not be started in the reading, arithmetic and writing demands of school until he or she is at least seven or eight years old. And his bias is not unshared—witness the upcoming text by David Elkind, "The Hurried Child."

Looking around in his community for a suitable place to share his views on child development, while at the same time building his practice in child counseling, he turned to the private schools. He personally visited every school in a two county radius, presenting his argument, and asking if they might want to consider instituting a "Readiness Test Program" at their pre-school. He offered to supply carefully prepared literature that the school could send home to all parents, explaining the "hazards" of sending their little Johnny or Suzie to the first grade too early. Then, in the same literature the parent would find a sign-up form to schedule Johnny or Suzie for Readiness Testing. After the testing, the parents would receive a detailed report with recommendations. Along with the report he would also send home information and brochures of various professional services, training sessions and seminars that he offered through his office. At the end of each term he also offered to see all interested parents in a group at the school to answer any questions they might have about the testing or about little Johnny or Suzie's future plans.

At present he has signed up most of the medium to large pre-schools in one county in Southern California, charging $35 per child tested. He has a team of retired credentialed school teachers and interns go out to the schools to administer the test for him. But the real "meat" of this idea lies in the spin-off services that he provides to those families whose children are tested.

We may not completely agree with his "hazardous" views of first grade horrors, but we must admire his ingenious business savvy!

Therapist Teaches Colleagues
How to Build a Consulting Business

One educational psychologist in Northern California became so successful in his own consulting services that he decided to share his know-how with his friends and "take it on the road."

It all began by teaching everyday personal skills such as communication, motivation, and leadership skills, to those whom he saw in group therapy. These groups became so popular that he decided to approach various companies in the area and propose a program of in-service training, teaching their employees these same skills. His consulting work became so profitable that he was forced to train other professionals to take over his groups at the office, and later, to conduct the in-service training programs for him. Realizing that most professionals in private practice are groping in the dark when it comes to getting started in outside consultation work, he decided to branch out to train mental health professionals in his methods, and teach them at the same time the business know-how in establishing consultation clientele.

In his "Adventures in ―――――" seminars, topics of training include, "Goal Setting, Leadership, Motivation, Effective Communication, Human Relations, Positive Attitudes, Personality, Self-Confidence, and Self-Management."

The training cost is $125 and is "structured into 20 modular units lasting 90 minutes each...can be taught in any schedule (evenings, weekends, etc.)...available in 18 countries and 8 languages. Over 87,000 people experienced it last year making it the number one human relations program in America." Not a bad track record from a skill that most of us already have but that we apply with only one or perhaps seven or eight at a time.

How does the old expression go?—"If you're going to fly with the eagles, quit hanging around with the turkeys!" *AIM HIGH!*

Successful Psychologist Has Good Advice
for Getting Referrals from the Religious Community

DeLoss ("Dee") Friesen dreamed about having his own successful practice while teaching at the University level for twelve long years. Finally, when the "system" was about to send him over the edge, he made the break, moved to Beaverton, Oregon, and today he has a flourishing practice, working with his wife, Ruby.

Dr. Friesen focused much of his practice-building efforts in courting the local religious leaders, and as a result, has a steady stream of referrals from these overworked men. We asked him if he would share some practical nuts-&-bolts advice about how to woo this valuable source of referrals. Here are his pointers:

"You have to face one fact of life in reaching out to ministers in your area: namely, most ministers have already been contacted by several psychotherapists wanting their referrals. But how many youth leaders and youth pastors have been contacted? This also would include church youth groups, community youth programs, YMCAs, Scout leaders (even den mothers!).

You can be more competitive with this group of religious leaders if you offer a skill that the therapists in your area do not seem to possess. Perhaps some additional training in marital communication, hypnosis, neuro-linguistic programming, neurological assessment or specialized work in working with suicidal patients, chronic depressives, rebellious adolescents, and so forth. Then, as you become acquainted with this potential referral source, you make sure this specialized skill is highlighted to him; perhaps summarizing some interesting cases to peak his interest.

Having something in common or of particular interest to the religious referral source is often an open door to good referrals. You have to face one thing though—if religious things are unimportant to you, he will most certainly refer to other more religiously-oriented therapists who have contacted his church in the past. But if you have any religious background, use that in presenting yourself to the religious community. It's not necessary that you come out of the identical religious background as he does. Most religious referral sources are simply concerned that you are sensitive to spiritual things, not so much that you share their identical belief system.

In terms of a common bond: If you have had some tragedy in your life, use that as an opening for certain groups. Someone who has gone through a divorce "appears" to have greater understanding of the pain involved in the process than someone who hasn't. A therapist coping with a stepchild situation "appears" to have a better handle on working with step-parents and step-children than someone not having gone through such things. If you have a retarded child or a physical disability in the family it can be useful. Membership in certain charitable organizations in the community can also give you an important "in" with the local religious referral source."

Excellent advice indeed! To this we would only add one footnote. In your ongoing involvements with church leaders, go out of your way to *Give Service!* For example: What's one major problem the minister faces at least once each year?—Who's going to fill in for him while he's on vacation? Many pastors are eager to have a mental health professional, who also has some spiritual interests, take a service or series of services for him, dealing with some practical issue of personal or family enrichment. They also welcome the professional running workshops or meetings at camps or retreats, singles and couples groups, or youth camps. Some professional clinicians are even running training classes in "How to Counsel Your Friends," "How to Improve Communication in Marriage," "How to Cope With the Problem Drinker," "Overcoming Stress," and "New Beginnings for Widows." Of course, this list could go on, ad infinitum.

And if the religious leader needs consultation by phone, give it willingly. You might also offer to see some of his congregation without charge if they are unable to afford treatment. This suggestion is about as popular as the Hong Kong flu, but you'd be surprised how many paying referrals can be generated by a few gratis sessions.

"Cancer Therapy" Seminars:
A Resounding Success For Psychotherapists

While research desparately struggles to find a cure for cancer in the laboratory, new research is showing the relationship between "emotional and mental states" and this disease. A group of health care professionals in Texas, including psychotherapists, have found tremendous acceptance across disciplinary lines for their research and treatment modalities for the cancer patient.

Here's a brief description from their seminar literature outlining Phase I of their seminar series:

"The Phase I Workshop introduces participants to the basic beliefs of ————'s approach to the emotional aspects of the cancer patient, including the concept and supporting research that the psyche and emotions participate in the development of cancer, and hold a valuable key in the treatment of the disease. It will involve participants in an experiential session. . ."

They describe their methods as "combining approved standard medical procedures with psychotherapy and a relaxation/visual imagery technique." Perhaps you have read or seen news reports from the publicity this group has received—there's that word again!

Last year this group of professionals held their three-day seminars in Boston, Seattle, New York City, San Diego, Dallas and St. Croix, and, get this—at $250 per participant!

In addition to the educational experience at the seminar, each professional who attends has the opportunity to purchase the group's text on the subject, and is informed of continuing education courses that they can take at the Texas Center for an additional tuition fee.

And guess how this whole thing got started? Simply as an outgrowth of their private practice in a Texas city, specializing in work with the "terminally ill" cancer patient. And even then, that practice was no slouch financially, you can be sure of that! But the seminar for professionals became so much in demand that they have had to delegate their patient-consultation to trainees.

How many people in your own family or circle of friends do you know who have died of cancer in the past few years? It has touched nearly every life today. If there was ever an area that was wide open for the mental health professional to specialize, this is it. Perhaps their training program could put you on the road to opening such a clinic— or even a training center—in your community. And don't forget the old truism: "All creativity and prosperity begins with *imitation*." Or perhaps you can apply your skills to some other area that has baffled medical (or some other) science, and that continues to plague mankind. And if you do, please share it with us for publication in upcoming editions of this manual.

You Can't Go Wrong With This One
In the '80's—Stress Management

The other day while having a parking lot ticket validated at the information desk at one of Southern California's largest hospitals, a stack of attractively produced brochures caught my eye. Let me share the major portions of it with you—it may suggest some possibilities in your area. The Title read:

STRESS MANAGEMENT. . . .Current Implications for
Prevention and Remediation Programs
A CONFERENCE FOR
HEALTH SERVICE PROVIDERS

Under this headline it goes on to describe the location of the conference, in the hospital itself.

The goal of the meeting is described as follows: "to present some useful and practical techniques for relief of stresses that can be integrated into daily practice." Four psychiatrists and two psychologists are listed as guest speakers, then the program schedule is laid out. It is interesting to note that in addition to listing each speaker's university affiliation, *and noting his private practice,* their published books are also described. And perhaps you already know that the book tables at workshops and conferences do a pretty good business!

On another page of this well-done brochure you find a section pointing out that one can get "Continuing Education Credit" for attending this conference, and listing all professions that qualify for such credit. Then we find the conference fee, and after taking a deep breath and sitting down, we are stunned to find that it's only $50! A conference or seminar or workshop these days in the two-digit category is a vanishing breed, isn't it? Why the "free lunch"?. . . .

We find in taking a look at the next section, titled, "Tax Deduction" the following reason for the "free lunch"—

"Treasury regulations permit an income tax deduction for educational expenses undertaken to maintain and improve professional skills.

Sponsored in part by a grant from Roche Laboratories. Any net proceeds which may accrue from the Conference will be contributed to the Psychiatric Clinic for Youth Endowment Fund charitable trust."

That's why the break in cost; the grant, and the donation plan. Now we're not trying to make you top-notch brochure copywriters—but if we give you a few lessons here and there, all the better. But when you do decide to put together some sort of seminar or workshop, get out this manual and look over these features again; they are potent advertising tools. Note the fee plus private grant plus charity angle!

Now our real purpose here is to help saturate your brain with ideas that have proven successful in building profitable mental health practices for those imaginative souls who have dreamed them up. How did these psychiatrists and psychologists benefit from this meeting? Certainly they did not pay this month's yacht payment from their Conference remuneration, did they? As we mentioned above, book sales were healthy at the Conference, and remember the mention of their practices? Well, even though they used the Conference to teach health care professionals the techniques for stress reduction, most professionals did not leave that meeting confident in doing it themselves with their own patients—or, they simply did not have the time. So, take a wild guess. . . .Where do you suppose they referred many of their patients who could profit from Stress Management Therapy? You're right on target again! The appointment books of most of the presenters on that Conference faculty showed evidence in black and white of the result of "giving" their time away for a "good cause." And royalties on those books?—They paid this month's slip fee for that yacht!—and then some!

Now don't get me wrong. . . .we're not implying that these men and women shared their expertise at the Conference simply to rake in Federal Reserve Notes; not at all! But since their practices demonstrated concrete growth in terms of patient referrals as a direct result of this activity, let's not pass over too quickly a strategy that achieves our primary goal—establishing successful practices.

In the '60's it was called "nerves" or "nervous disorders." In the '70's it was called "anxiety states" or "acute anxiety attacks." Now, in the '80's it's called "stress" and "stress burnout." You'll find these new handles for old enemies cropping up in almost every major popular magazine and tabloid. Mr. and Mrs. Citizen is now more informed than ever, and they are accepting the fact that emotional factors (stress) contribute to many of their headaches; literally and figuratively.

There's the old addage: "An idea whose time has come." Well, it seems that you are licensed to practice in a Profession whose time has come! You can't go wrong with this one in the '80's!

Double Your Rate of Monthly Referrals
By Using a Technique Pioneered By a Dentist

You wouldn't think we as mental health professionals could learn much from observing the tactics a west coast dentist used to double his rate of monthly patient referrals, would you? Ahh—you might be surprised; have a look see at this powerful idea. . . .

On the west coast, as elsewhere in this country, there are too many dentists coming out of dental school, and too few mouths that need fixing. Many dentists now, even after years of flourishing practices, are complaining about empty waiting rooms and are forced to "moonlight" to make ends meet. However, one group of business-wise D.D.S.'s in California have found a way to keep many mouths asking for appointments on the phone to their offices. What's their method?

A monthly Newsletter. That's their method, and it works wonders! The title of the Newsletter, which is sent to hundreds of local residents, is called "ROOTS—Or 'Where Your Dentist Is Coming From. . .'" Under "ROOTS" you find a photo of a dentist and his pretty dental assistant tenderly working on the mouth of a young teenager. The teen has a nice big smile on his face and under the picture the headline, "Nice smiles happen at CDB." CDB stands for "Childrens' Dental Building" the practice DBA, fictitious name. Under this heading one of the center's orthodontists is described, with his impressive experience and credentials. Then the article goes into "the treatment of crooked teeth. . ." and explains what happens on a first visit. We just start to get hooked by the drama of this article when we are referred to page three, inside, as we are in a daily newspaper. The interesting article concludes by warning parents that the earlier they get their little ones in for an exam the better able to save money in future dental problems. And a beautiful last finishing touch, the article concludes, "Dr. ——— also treats adult patients—you're never too old to correct the appearance of teeth you don't like!" See why they double their patient referrals?!

Getting back to the front page of our Newsletter: Alongside the photo is another headline; "Insurance—How you can help yourself." Now there's a great attention getter! The thrust of this article is to first explain how to fill out the average policy, the misconception of the 100% coverage, and other practical tips. The article also concludes on page three with a provocative checklist of what to watch for when dealing with an unscrupulous D.D.S. Just the mentioning of such things would tend to give the reader greater confidence in CDB, wouldn't it?

I won't tax your patience with too much details here, but perhaps you might like a quickie overview of the rest of the Newsletter, in case you see the potential for your own purposes. On page two we find "Notes From The Director," a personal letter describing why CDB's fees are so much lower than other dental offices (because of patient volume); ("our office stays open 7-days, a total of 66 hours a week...Our group wants you to have more dental care and health for your dollar"). Now watch this one—the practice director closes his very convincing letter with this commanding clincher; "I'm asking you personally to tell one friend, relative, or co-worker to call our office and benefit from our good management. Don't let me down—I won't let you down." and he bids us farewell with this—

Brush and Floss!

Donald M. ————, D.D.S.

On the same page is an interesting article about "What the Different 'dontics' mean"; a small box advertising for a dental assistant because the practice is "so busy and growing so fast." The next page contains some useful medical information on "Patient Rights" and a small section, "We speak your language," pointing out that "Our staff is experienced with Spanish, Portuguese, Philippino, Japanese, Chinese, Vietnamese, Persian, and sign language. We're here to help!" If I had the slightest hint of a toothache, how could I possibly resist?

Now on the back, here's the key motivator: In big, white on black letters, we read, "WILL THE DENTIST LISTEN?" followed by a heart-rending story of a woman who had a terrible experience in a dental chair as a child and her fear that the dentist will not understand. Under this, in equally bold type the words, "WE CAN'T LISTEN IF YOU

DON'T CALL. . ." And if that weren't enough to soothe our fears, the Newsletter ends with, "YOU TOO CAN BE BRAVE"—offering to give every kid the 'BRAVERY PILL,' a muscle relaxant to make local anesthesia easier. Sensational, isn't it!

And it doubles the normal rate of monthly patient referrals to the traditional dentist. But what about your practice? If a dentist with not much exciting to work with can come up with something this captivating with dental news, what about us clinical types, who deal in the raw material of the best soap opera every day, day in, day out? A monthly or bi-monthly newsletter reporting on unusual breakthroughs with cases; interviews with patients with unusual stories who have overcome some kind of habitual behavior or obsession; "How To" advice from you about some topic of interest to many laymen today; reports of your own or others' research into interesting problems (for example, the cancer therapy); reports on what one can learn from various psychological tests about himself or his marriage; an ongoing analysis of the various characters in the soaps from a professional's point of view; offer of a free evaluation just prior to the opening of school for readiness or adjustment assessment; and perhaps a regular Question and Answer Section to round it all out. Now this list could go on forever; but I think you get the picture. . . .Not only would the Newsletter notion bring in many new faces, but it would be just plain fun to do, if you like to write and are good at the art of plain talk. For the latter I recommend with great enthusiasm Rudolph Flesch's classic work, *The Art of Plain Talk* published by Collier Books.

Why do so many people buy the *National Enquirer?* We tend to look down our professional noses at it, don't we? But people love it! Next time you're at the supermarket, pick up a copy (force yourself!), examine carefully how the articles are written, how intriguing the headlines are, and the way the stories get curiosity stirred up. Gear your newsletter in this direction, making it "Newsy"—and your tax bracket will tell the REAL story!

How One Therapist Built a Prosperous Part-Time Practice By Overcoming the "Stigma" of Therapy

The child or teenager with problems is not unusual or rare when he or she refuses to be "drug into a shrink's office" for help because "the kids'll think I'm nuts, or somethin'." And although mental health services are finding more favor these days, when it comes to therapy for their kids, many parents share the shrink-stigma with their offspring. But they both need help, so, what to do?

One therapist who has a magic touch with kids found the way to overcome the effects of the stigma for both parents and children. He's a licensed Child Therapist, a licensed Educational Psychologist, AND he loves to help kids do their homework! That's the key! He has combined his talents in counseling with his liking for *tutoring*.

So in promoting his practice, he leans heavily on the need problem children have for tutorial help. Because of their emotional and interpersonal problems, he explains, these children fall down in their studies, are treated as failures by their teachers, and mess up their future careers in the process. What does he offer?

He offers to see the children or teens as their tutor first-off. When he wins their confidence and trust, which doesn't take long, he may persuade them to take some "neat" tests and perhaps let Mom and Dad come in and join their sessions. Before you know it, not only are Junior's grades and report cards showing good signs of progress, but family strife and other difficulties are getting direct intervention.

Using this strategic approach many kids are reached and helped who otherwise would never have found their way into the consultation room. But this flexible therapist helped them and their parents neutralize the sting of the stigma. Ever wondered why they give you free samples of cheese and various delicacies at the markets? It's simple: After you've tried the free sample, that makes it much easier for you to go the next harder step of spending that $2.59 for the real thing! This therapist is simply a good clinician, and a fine business man.

Is There Room In Your Practice
For the Greatest Tragedy of All?

There is no hurt greater than this one. Here are the words of a patient who got help, and talks about the hurt:

"It's not a recent experience, but it's the crippling kind that you never forget. . .The doctor who was on call had never seen me before. He was very brutal and blunt. That doctor came in and said, 'Your baby will be born today and will probably not survive.

Then he turned and left the room. John Paul, Jr. was born dead. . . .

After that I needed to talk. I found myself repeating the same things over and over again, even telling strangers on the bus about losing my baby. I'd practically drag people in off the street to listen to me. . ."

This woman and her husband suffered the greatest tragedy—losing your own child. Once the medical personnel in the hospital did all they could to save the baby, the couple was left, high and dry, all alone, not even a social worker to comfort or assist them.

This couple is not alone in their suffering. Hundreds of families are experiencing this catastrophe every day. To assist such parents, and professionals who must deal with them, a volunteer organization has been formed—it's called AMEND; Aiding Mothers Experiencing Neonatal Death. Nation-wide this group of lay counselors helps the grieving parents bear their new cross and pick up the pieces to begin anew.

Did you know about this group? If you are concerned and want to help ease their pain, you might consider contacting AMEND. You can offer your services to their parents—they make direct referrals after AMEND begins the initial grief preparation work. If you don't feel qualified in dealing with this heavy business (may you never qualify through first hand experience) AMEND will provide training to get you ready to help. A hospital social worker can get you in touch with AMEND.

Planned Parenthood Adjustment Counseling— A New Opportunity for the Psychotherapist

One imaginative Marriage, Family and Child Therapist in Oregon found a new channel for her talents. A personal friend worked as a lay counselor at a local Planned Parenthood Clinic. As they talked, she became more convinced that her skills in Marital Counseling could be invaluable at the clinic.

She asked more questions than an FBI investigator to pinpoint the best way to go about presenting her ideas to the clinic director. When she had carefully planned her presentation, she went to see him personally.

She wisely had her presentation well organized and typed out for the director to refer to as they talked about her new brainchild and how it could benefit the clinic's services to their patients.

Basically, she proposed that the clinic hire her as their professional mental health consultant. She would work with those women who (1) find out they are pregnant and don't want to be, (2) the parents of these women, (3) women and their partners who are considering the serious effects of choosing an abortion as their answer, and (4) those couples lost in confusion about the ramifications of sterilization and vasectomy.

In her proposed position, she offered, at no cost to the clinic, to lease video taping equipment from the university where she had affiliation, and to tape interviews with women and couples who have made good adjustments. This could be a powerful counseling and adjustment film series to help her, and the other staff, deal with these difficult problems in their patients.

The results? She is now kept so busy that she must divide her time between her booming practice and her consulting work—practicing what she preached in her proposal!

Got any possibilities in your world?

Recently we got a request from a reader asking to purchase another copy of the *Handbook*. As it turned out, she had loaned her first copy to a friend, and you know the rest of this story. . . .she never saw it again.

While chatting with her I asked if she had come up with any new twists and practical ideas for making her fairly new practice "fly." She and a partner began a year or so ago in Marriage Therapy, naming their practice, "The Growing Tree." She reported excellent growth in this short time, having implemented many of the techniques in this manual. Then she described a new venture which she has begun and reported preliminary signs of success. Here's her report paraphrased:

A few months ago I looked into our local Chamber of Commerce for the possibility of getting our practice some good recognition here. They hold what is called, "Chamber Mixers" each month or so. In these Mixers all the local business and professional people in the area who belong get together to chit chat, talk about their respective businesses, and swap business cards. I did the same thing and people really seemed interested in our work.

Before the next Mixer I came up with a new idea. So I put together a Certificate that I could hand out to those I met at the Mixer. This Certificate entitled anyone to a free initial consultation, for either an adult, teen or child. They were really well received there when I gave them out. No way to know just yet what the outcome will be, it's much too soon.

This idea has merit, doesn't it? Of course, she put together a really good certificate, making it professional and in very good taste—nothing sleazy about it. If it did not have the professional touch, it would likely do little good in generating referrals. The verdict on its effectiveness?—We'll wait to hear from her—and from *you!*

Marriage Encounter Works!
A Way to Make It Work for Your Practice

Who hasn't heard about, or seen a satisfied customer proudly displaying his or her or their bumper sticker, or seen a new glow on a patient's face who has just come back from a Marriage Encounter weekend retreat? It all started in the Catholic Church, and the methods have proven so effective in making basically healthy marriages healthier, that it spread like wild-fire throughout almost every other denomination in the church. Even the Jewish community now sponsors Encounters out of their synagogues.

The reason for their effectiveness? They have simply applied some basic techniques of written communication to overcome the defensiveness and fear created by verbal non-communication. But no need to go into the ins and outs of their methods—they are open to anyone or any married couple, who would attend an Encounter weekend (that is, if you don't mind waiting about a year to get the opportunity!).

During the past few years a few bright Therapists in different parts of the same state saw that *here* was an idea whose time had indeed come. They asked themselves, "Why should people have to wait a year to get this kind of blessing in their marriage? I have all the skill and know-how to provide the same week-end experiences. I don't have a church, but do I really need one or even a church affiliation?" Unlike many dreamers, this clinician put some action and foot leather where his dreams had been. He began the nation-wide organization "Marriage Enrichment," which has grown so fast that, guess what?—You now have to wait a year to attend! He's produced many books, tapes, seminars and public appearances as spin-offs from this work as well. But because his first love is college teaching and private practice, he has trained qualified MFCC's and lay-counselors to run the Enrichment weekends and followup groups.

The other man, a clinical psychologist, began a similar venture out of his own church. This church is a non-denominational and huge church in a heavily populated area. But because of their maverick, no-denomination-connection status, they had no way into the Marriage Encounter system. But, as most entrepreneurs will tell you, every dark cloud has that silver lining!

Although he had a lively private practice—getting ample and steady referrals from the church—and although he enjoyed various classes he taught at the church, he *made time* to put his own dreams into action. With the pastor's blessing he formed the twin brother to Marriage Encounter, borrowing liberally from its philosophy and technique bag of tricks, and called it "Enjoying Marriage." Well folks, it grew so fast that every weekend for months is booked solid. He has since parted company with the church affiliation, running the Enjoying Marriage program out of his practice itself. This retreat is a bit different from both of the above, in that it has a strong appeal to born-again Christians, and uses the Bible almost entirely along with the other methods described earlier. And that is precisely what makes this experience so effective and so much in demand.

Too often we look at a successful program, like the Marriage Encounter movement, and we kick our professional ego's for not coming up with such a "brilliant" idea ourselves. That's hard on the egos. . . .they get enough kicking from others! Wouldn't it be wiser to take a look at those super-colossal-smash-successes and fiddle around with them in our mind; like the Rubik's Cube puzzle, until we come up with an "Ah-ha!" modification or just something a little bit new in order that we might undertake our own smash hit? That's where successes, the really big ones, are made, in the final analysis: Not in something brand new that has never existed before. But someone has simply taken something common-place and said, "I wonder what would happen if I took this and put it over here. . . .and added a touch of this. . . .and suppose we remove this and. . . ." etc., etc. After all, that's the way most psychotrophic drugs are discovered; that's the way biofeedback found its entrance into our offices; and if you will dust off your copy of *The Ego And The Id* up there on your bookshelf, you will discover that that's the way Freud started the whole thing!

Here's a little exercise to help you stretch your creativity:

(1) List three unorthodox and novel ways that you could use in treating agoraphobic patients using methods proven effective in related problems:

Idea 1: _____

Idea 2: _____

Idea 3: _____

(2) The biggest epidemics in this country today are the "runaway wives" and the "men in mid-life crisis." List below three treatment approaches to these problems that combine techniques used for years successfully with other disorders:

Idea 1: _____

Idea 2: _____

Idea 3: _____

Now if you're tempted to skip this little exercise and read on, as most of us would be, remember this—you spent a bundle on this manual, right? Don't cheat yourself out of an important opportunity to discover how ingenious and inventive you really are! The kind of mental processes that this task requires are the precise mental tools that you will need to refine if your practice is ever to become more than mediocre. Why not go back and give it another shot?

BEFORE AND AFTER:
<u>Before</u>—**An Average of One New Referral Every Three Weeks.**
<u>After</u>—**A Two-Week Waiting List: What Made The Difference?**

In a nutshell—SPECIALIZATION.

In the San Fernando Valley, a bedroom community just north of Los Angeles, a partnership of three MFCC's and Clinical Social Workers tried for several years to build a practice that would support their champagne tastes. After many well intended attempts to get those Valley residents to notice their many skills, they had to settle for beer!

However, one key decision and a change in emphasis with a narrowed focus did the trick and brought on the champagne.

Realizing that they were competing with literally hundreds of other equally qualified therapists in their area, they decided to specialize. Specialize in what? Using the popular womens' magazines and tabloids they surveyed what the average American woman was most concerned about these days. Their finding—the "housewife's syndrome," or as we say in the bizz, "agoraphobia."

They discarded their Ho-Hum clinic name and zeroed in on this one problem in their name itself. Then they had brochures printed up that defined the illness, gave some interesting stories about its victims, and reported some findings of recent behavior therapy and biofeedback research. Next they described their treatment "staff" and their "innovative methods" for treating the agoraphobic patient successfully (they had actual cases from previous work to report true results). They even inserted a testimonial from an actual patient as to her "new life" since discovering this Center.

Next came a series of promotions and news releases to the Los Angeles media—arranged by a skillful PR agency. This resulted in TV exposure on the 6 o'clock news under the heading "health and science news." You can predict what happened!

Our physician colleagues discovered the many benefits of narrowing the focus, then dentists followed suit, then attorneys began to specialize. Try this little experiment if your practice needs some new life. Spend this coming Saturday afternoon in the local public library. Pass up the section you're used to sniffing around and sit down with some of those magazines that you never read but keep in your waiting room for others. Take notes. Look for trends. Fads. Topics for the advice columnists. And don't forget *Reader's Digest!* After this little research adventure, look for the common thread that runs through several of the most popular soaps and TV series.

Can you or someone you hire and train provide a service to your community to help deal with this problem which is on the minds of thousands of Americans every day? *The Waiting List awaits!*

Therapist-Pilot Uses His Love of Flying To Build Lucrative "Treatment Seminars" for Phobics

When you sit down to consult with someone who wants to build a new business from scratch, or someone who wants to specialize in his or her own practice to generate more referrals, the first thing you look for is the "first love." What does he or she love to do when relaxing? How would they spend their time just enjoying life if they could do anything under the sun they wished? Then, to assure a greater probability of success in the business or practice, you attempt to work that interest, that "first love" into the operation, even if only by analogy, or in symbolic form.

You might wonder if this is not carrying the notion of building a profitable practice too far. But one behavioral therapist recently showed us how it was done—and done so well that there's now a heavy demand for his "first love" therapy.

Using first-rate public relations methods, this therapist in Newport Beach, California was able to tell some 1,234,114 people about his new work. Of them, thousands suffer from the very problem that he treats—aerophobia, the fear of flying. Here's a sample from his story from the *Los Angeles Times,* January 24, 1982. . . .

"Your flight for Europe leaves in the morning—and you're uneasy. . . .You have an extra drink to help you sleep. Maybe two. The fear of flying. . . .By the time you board the plane you're a nervous wreck. Determined to go through with the flight in spite of every nerve in your body resisting your conscious decision. Sound familiar? Well, it is for legions of travelers. Fear of flying, aerophobia, afflicts millions. . . .

However, those who want to overcome their fear of flying can be helped, according to Glen H. ———— of Newport Beach who heads *ThAIRapy,* a fear-of-flying treatment program. ———— is a licensed commercial pilot with 20 years of flying experience and he's a behavioral therapist who's done individual and family counseling for 12 years.

'You can't be afraid if you're relaxed,' ———— says. . . .

This interesting article proceedes to explain his method of treatment; basically, he uses a progressive relaxation, systematic desensitization and cognitive modality, helping his clients learn how to relax themselves, and getting familiar with how one of those big monsters get off the ground.

After describing in very general terms these procedures, this therapist gives his readers some "free" advice on how they can handle their flying jitters—good, practical ideas. Remember this tip: When you put out a News Release and then are interviewed, or you write your own article, be sure to GIVE OUT FREE, SELF-HELP INFOR-MATION. This significantly increases the probability that your article will make it into print.

After the free tips, the writer informs us how much the treatment seminars cost—

"———— has several programs to help the aerophobic: on an individual basis, in five to eight sessions over a two-month period (costing about $500); in six-week workshops with a few other people (365); a single four-hour evening seminar $15; and a 'relaxation cassette tape' ($12.95) to be used in conjunction with one of the programs, or even by itself without the rest of the instruction."

Look at the choices! This therapist has used his head, hasn't he? And note the offer of a cassette at the end. Undoubtedly he'll get a flood of orders for that cassette from people that he'll never see in his office. The cassette, self-help, self-education business (and including the video recording market) is the next giant boom to watch in promoting your practice.

Then after a string of testimonials from happy non-phobics, watch how the article builds this therapist's credibility and gives him a personal touch to help the reader feel comfortable in picking up the phone to call his office for an appointment. . . .

"'You can develop a new way of relating to flying.' ———— should know. His hobby is aerobatics (trick flying). 'I enjoy the union with the plane,' he said. Now there's a man who really enjoys flying.

ThAIRapy is at 1234 Ocean Drive, Suite 123, Newport Beach, phone (714) 222-3333.'"

From this short exerpt you get a feel for the power of this media in bringing in new patients, don't you? It's a good idea to keep in mind when instructing your PR person, or in doing your own promotions, to give yourself, your practice, and your work a PERSONALITY. Make your practice easy to approach. Structure the article so that after the reader puts it down most of his questions are answered, his interest is stirred, his needs or hurts have been clearly defined, he feels that you are "just what I've been looking for," and, he knows how to get in touch with you.

We can't stress too much the importance of knowing how to use the press release in generating public interest in you and your work. And the cost? ZIP!

How One Clinician Got Her Name
In the Referral Resource Guide of a Local Hotline

The therapist we refer to here did not even know that her city had an emergency hot line until she stumbled onto a small news article in one of those throw-aways. The article simple described one of the Hotline's volunteers who had spent "thousands of hours" checking out various community professionals that they could use to refer callers to for counseling. "I've been in this town and am listed in the phone book for the last six years" she thought to herself "and yet they didn't call me....how come?" Realizing that was a locking-the-barn-door-after-the-horse-got-out question, she quit feeling sorry for herself and got down to real business.

"What can I do NOW, now that I know that they exist; what can I do now to let them know that I exist?" Now that little question is more like it! Here's the plan she came up with....

She typed out a short note to the manager of the Hotline whose name was mentioned in the article. In the note she simply said that she had seen the news release and that she was glad to learn that their service was so near, since she had been referring her own after-hour calls to the Suicide Prevention Center some 35 miles away. She then said that she would call her early the following week to discuss their services. Note here that she said, to discuss *their* services, NOT hers! Now, of course, there's nothing whatever wrong with calling to tell them about your services. You can even drop them a short blurb about your practice specialization, giving details about how they can use you as a referral resource, if they would like. And that method does get results. But some therapists are more reluctant to come right out and ask for this. So the method this therapist chose to employ may be the back door approach, but it is a potent one indeed.

When she called the following week she asked many questions about the Hotline staff, how they were trained, hours in service, how they handled suicidal calls, etc. When she told the manager that she would put their number on her answering service for use for her own patients, then *the manager asked some questions about her!*

The therapist had a golden opportunity to describe her near-by practice in detail. To her surprise, she asked if perhaps she would consider "serving on our board of directors" and perhaps "you wouldn't mind coming over to one of our monthly in-service training sessions and teaching our volunteers about how to deal with particular cases."

Her after-hour callers no longer had to call a distant number when they couldn't reach her, and, using the tangential approach, she initiated a successful new relationship. This same approach is effective in making contact with many auxilliary mental health services in your area. The "letter-first, then call" strategy you will note is used by many therapists we have described. Why? Because to make the maximal impact on someone who has never heard of you, you need repetition of the message. And the message is YOU. We might go one step further in this regard: After sending the short note, then making the friendly information gathering call, follow that up with one more "thank you" oriented letter. One, Two, Three! And perhaps in the second letter you might say that in a few days you will send along a brochure describing the services available at your office. One, Two, Three, Four! How did we learn that three times three equals nine? Repetition. How does an unknown therapist become—"Oh yes, I know just the therapist to refer them to, Dr. ————, her office is just across town, and I know she handles that problem"? Repetition.

Workman's Comp—A Rich Referral Source

Dr. B———— had never done very much in the way of outside consultation, restricting himself primarily to one-to-one consultation with his own patients. However, he had begun exploring ways to increase his practice and was mentally ready for something "new." He had already enlisted the help of an educational psychologist to work in his office so that he could routinely test all new patients as part of their initial intake procedure.

One day he was working with a new widow patient, helping her in her grief. She brought up the fact that she was considering filing workman's compensation suit because stress on the job had killed her husband. As he talked with her it dawned on him that he could help her in dealing with her attorney, provide psychological input to the case, and, make an important contact with a workman's comp attorney in the process. He got her consent and called the attorney.

As he talked with the attorney he tried to go out of his way to give information that would help the attorney help her (and his own commission in the case), and then added; "By the way, did you know that we have in our office a psychologist that specializes in diagnostics, including brain dysfunction and brain damage. He's a wiz with the Halsted-Reitan Battery, a neurological test. . ." Before they ended their little talk, he had established a working relationship with this busy attorney, and told him that "I'll put some information about the Reitan Battery in the mail for you in the next couple of days; I think you'll find it interesting." He asked his psychologist to prepare a one-page fact sheet on the Reitan, with the emphasis, of course, on brain injured patients and the reliability of this instrument. Along with this promised information he attached his business card and a friendly letter, saying how much he enjoyed talking with the attorney the other day.

In Chapter 7 we discussed the Pyramiding Effect, remember? Here's a perfect example of how one practitioner used it to help the patient, and get some good practice exposure at the same time. Are you missing some good bets during caseload review? During intake screening? At the time of termination? Try this just for practice: When you see your next patient in consultation, on their chart write the name of at least *one* professional person in that patient's life that you can find some good reason to contact. Then, when you have their name and the patient's consent, enter in your appointment book: "Practice Promotion Time" or "Practice Development Time." Under this heading, write the name and number or address. Then on that day and hour, go into action. And if you don't write it down, it will remain a good intention and will never get done.

Perhaps you would like to close this manual here and take a look at a chart or two???

Therapist Uses Her Teaching Know-How
To Promote Her Home-Office Practice

In a recent telephone interview with Susan Forthman, M.A., an MFCC in Southern California, Sue reports that she has generated four new patients in a short period of time by means of her teaching—not counseling—abilities. Here's a paraphrased recap of that interview:

"Here in the San Fernando Valley we have what is called a "Free University"* called the *Learning Tree*. They offer inexpensive classes in such things as: Making Money in Mail Order; Dance; Art; Photography; Yoga; and classes in practical self-help subjects. A few months ago I started teaching a class called 'Depression, Blues and the Blahs.' It's a good sized class and since then I've gotten four new clients from this class. I have also gotten clients from my class called 'Overcoming Anxiety.' This is really an excellent way to become known. Also, many people check you out in the class to see what kind of a therapist you are, whereas they wouldn't come in for an appointment in therapy first."

She goes on to say that she has special announcements printed up describing the classes and giving the number of the *Learning Tree* for more information. She then sends these announcements to. . . .

". . .my present clients, my old clients, various other therapists I know, and even my old professors. I also send out news releases. I get a pretty good response in terms of new clients this way. I have even taken a stack of these announcements to my beauty shop and the owner lets me leave them there. I got one call saying, 'I'm not interested in your course, but how much do you charge for therapy?'."

We concluded the interview with her account of an amusing story of how her love for garage sales turned into new business in her practice. . . .

"I had just made the rounds at a nearby garage sale and bought a few things. Before I left I asked the gal running the sale if she might be interested in attending my class—as I pulled out my announcement. When she showed interest in it, I asked if I might leave some for others there on her card table. She not only agreed, but she said to me, 'Do you give talks?. . .I am the program director of Parents Without Partners and we need

---

*Another clinician teaches at her city's Recreation Department to bring in new business.

someone for February 6th; could you come over and give a talk
to the members?'"

Many professionals would say that Susan was just plain lucky. But
someone has wisely defined *luck* this way:

Luck is when PREPARATION meets OPPORTUNITY!

How many of us are mentally set to promote our own practices even
when we are "killing time" shopping, or having our hair done, or
waiting around at the local garage, etc., etc.

We have to take off our hats to Sue—nice job of putting into action
some of the things she learned from the first edition of this *Handbook*
and some good business savvy in practice promotion.

Another Marriage and Family Therapist has used her teaching skills
at a local State University to generate new business. She teaches
counseling courses in the Educational Psychology Department and
reports that in nearly every class, she has someone come up to her
asking if she can see them in her office. She reports that she gets the
same type of question from students in her church classes that she
teaches at a large Baptist Church every Sunday evening, but there she
finds the rate of new patients even higher.

The story is told about a bright, young executive. He was full of
ambition and eager to make a name for himself. He worked for a
company just getting started in the fast-food business, selling hamburgers.

One day he burst into the president's office with what he thought
was a brilliant idea. "Let's set up a research department" he said "and
experiment until we find a way to make our hamburgers more
appealing to the man on the street."

The president set back in his chair patiently listening to this
"brilliant" idea. Then he got up, put on his overcoat and escorted his
young eager-beaver down the street to a local MacDonalds. There he
bought a Big Mac. Sitting at a nearby table he proceeded to open the
Big Mac and laid it in front of his wide-eyed genius. "Do you see that?"
he asked, "All the research we need is right in there!"

The lesson of this silly little story? When someone else has gone to
all the trouble of trying some fool idea and has found some measure of
success in it in their own enterprise, there's really no need for us to
rack our brains for another fool idea just so we can say we discovered
something brand new. You've just met some of those imaginative—

and brave—souls in the foregoing pages. You've not only been given their ideas, but you also have enough of their blueprints to do the job yourself.

After you do the job yourself, and perhaps add some creative twist to it from your own experience, and after you've done the field testing and collected the "results" data, we'll have another success story to report. . . .*YOURS!* And when you do, we'll be pleased to publish it for you (with credit due, of course) in the next edition!

With that invitation, we close this chapter, wishing you abundant success in filling that appointment book of yours. But before we forget, let us leave you with these words from some wise old owl—

"In order to make ends meet, you have to get off yours!"

CHAPTER TWELVE

A PERSONAL DISCOVERY

CHAPTER 12
A PERSONAL DISCOVERY

You and I could have ended this manual at the conclusion of the last chapter. If we had, you would have all the information, suggestions and "tips" needed to establish a lively and prosperous practice of your own.

But this Handbook was intended from its inception as something that might contribute meaningfully to the lives of those who read it. Having personally lived through the difficult period of building a practice from scratch, I wanted to help the newcomer over those rough spots—to serve as a kind of guide, as one who was familiar with the journey, the detours, and the scenic short-cuts. To the experienced "old timers" in the field I hoped to extend the hand of encouragement—to urge them on to expand their present practice and their conceptualization of what a practice can ultimately become.

If, in this Handbook, you have been guided, challenged, and encouraged, then I have successfully met my objectives. You have at your disposal the ingredients of a thriving professional practice.

But there is something missing yet. Something that acts as a key or catalyst, causing the ingredients to all work together for good to fulfill the recipe. If we had stopped at the last chapter I would have done you a disservice indeed.

Thus, by way of a personal account of my own experience I will complete the recipe for you. The Key or Catalyst that you will discover in this chapter will have a profound effect upon your professional life, your practice growth, and will surely influence *you* personally as well—as it did me.

For as long as I can remember my driving ambition was to climb to the pinnacle of academic excellence, to achieve all that I could in the intellectual community with a high degree of mastery. I suppose this ambition stemmed from the frustrations of a visual impairment from birth which kept me from excelling in more physical endeavors, i.e., football, baseball, tennis, etc. Legal blindness might keep me from the varsity, but I had a shot at the Ph.D.!

A doctorate in psychology became my magnificent obsession. Even as a Sophomore in College I knew, KNEW that someday I would achieve that measure that I had set for myself. And with equal assurance, I KNEW that it represented my ultimate fulfillment—like the itch that is finally scratched. Then, I assumed, after attaining that visionary goal, I could use whatever knowledge and skill I had accumulated along the way to serve man. And along with these mighty presuppositions went one additional belief; namely that in the process I would find personal and lasting peace of mind, satisfaction and fulfillment in life.

Well, the itch got scratched! After a short, two-year interruption between the masters and doctoral programs at which time I worked as a rehabilitation counselor, the work for the Ph.D. was resumed and completed. After "a pound of flesh" and two years battling the dissertation crusades, the magnificent obsession, the dream, the vision was a reality. For a while the thrill lasted. But something was wrong . . . something was missing. There was no lightening or thunder. The heavens did not part. There were no trumpets.

The thing that kept haunting my mind were the lyrics from that old song, "Is that all there is?" Is that all there is?

The itch again needed scratching!

Talk about an anti-climax! How could it be that half-a-lifetime's dream, now fulfilled in every sense, could not satisfy? How was it conceivable that the accomplishment of so great a burning desire could be so empty, so utterly hollow? Is that all there is?!

That's all there was. Just the completion of another step up the ladder. It was not unlike handing in that final term paper for any of scores of psychology classes along the way. And I don't even have to tell you that the doctorate did not have any peace of mind or intrinsic fulfillment attached to it. The thing that I thought promised true satisfaction and meaning turned out to be an empty victory.

Like the mirage for the thirsty man. Up ahead he sees a lush, green, and abundantly wet oasis calling to him. He runs, crawls and staggers along in the blazing sun, finally to reach the final dune. When he comes to the top of the dune he finds that it was all an illusion. His eyes—and his appetites—had played tricks on him. There's nothing there. It's gone. And worst of all, he's still thirsty!

Cognitive dissonance (and thirst) being what it is, the mind must find some way to adapt to its new position of disquiet. "Ah ha!" I cleverly told myself, "the fulfillment that you've been searching for will be found in serving mankind; using that Ph.D. for the good of humanity." New hope rose in my heart. All wasn't lost after all. All I need do now was to fling myself headlong into my work in psychotherapy with the same zeal that I pursued that degree on the wall and I would catch that illusive rainbow. So I did.

I poured over my journals. I attended workshops and conventions. I got an article published. I began experimenting with various modalities and treatment approaches and developing some innovations. I joined a professional association. Bev, my wife, and I sat around in our leisure time discussing counseling innovations and ideas, living our work day in and day out. Even on those rare vacations I would take my professional journals and "techniquey" books with me.

Then something strange began to happen. I began to notice that no matter what modality I used, no matter how clever or dramatic (or traditional) it might be, the patients all seemed to progress, or not to progress at about the same rate. "Surely" I told myself "Surely this new twist on that old analytical approach should increase therapeutic gain?" "Certainly the behavioristic methodology with its preciseness and objectivity will show greater results?" "Undoubtedly the gestalt-experiential approach with its genuineness and authenticity is the answer?" As the search went on I became increasingly cognizant that something was not right. Something was missing. My mirage was beginning to blur and dissolve away again.

What was taking place was that I was experiencing first hand the truth of the words from a classic paper by Hans Strupp on psychotherapy outcome. Strupp hit the nail on the head!

" . . . *all* forms of intervention designated as "therapy" appear to result in beneficial outcomes under *some* circumstances. Such 'intermittent reinforcements' bolster the therapist's belief that he is engaged in a worthwhile and socially useful activity."*

What was to me before only an extreme, if not outrageous, theoretical assertion now became living reality. My "belief was bolstered" certainly that I was engaged in a "socially useful" function. But as you might guess, that is little comfort for one as obsessive-compulsive as I.

---

*Hans H. Strupp, "Toward a Reformulation of the Psychotherapeutic Influence", *International Journal of Psychiatry*, 11, 1973, p. 269.

The itch, the emptiness, and the restlessness came roaring back with renewed fervor. And again the haunting lyrics, "Is that all there is?!" What next?

Throughout both undergraduate and graduate school another dream that held my fancy involved "someday" and "somehow" entering into my own professional private practice on a full time basis. From the first weeks following masters level work I had successfully conducted part-time practices—and loved the freedom and challenge of the enterprise. There was also a risk involved in the activity. Could I, through my own ingenuity and resourcefulness, build a lively practice and keep it growing? That was the risk, that was the challenge.

The challenge and the risk and the responsibility all combined to suggest to my restless soul that "Ah ha! this MUST BE the answer, THE WAY to scratch that infernal itch."

So off we went, Bev and I, full tilt, hurling ourselves 150% into the pursuit of a dream; our own full-time practice—she working with the little ones, the kids, and me treating the taller kids, the adults. We began by "fading in" gradually as I have recommended in this manual, first on a part-time basis. Then we decided that since the methods at practice development were proving out, we burned our first major bridge behind us so that we could not retreat, even out of panic. That involved turning down a well-paid job as psychologist at the local V.A. Hospital. A decision that was somewhat terrifying to say the least.

But cutting off that source of security proved to be a tremendous motivator to me. The risk, challenge and responsibility were now magnified and I had to make the practice support my family, car, home, put food on the table, etc., etc. And at the same time the emptiness and restlessness was passified: the pressure to survive kept me from noticing the void.

Time passed and through careful implementation of many of the strategies that you find in this Handbook, our practice became successful and the roller coaster began to level off. The furniture got paid off. The bills were finally all paid on time. And we reached the point of needing additional therapists to see our patients in outlying areas of the city.

A professional private practice with Bev and I working side by side on a full-time basis was no longer in the realm of fantasy. A dream was again fulfilled. But as you have doubtless already suspected, with the fulfillment of the dream came that old familiar unrest. The void in my life had only been temporarily appeased. Although the thirst had been quenched for a time, that insatiable longing for "something" was again at the door.

I can imagine your thoughts as you read this. You're probably saying, "Brother, this guy doesn't know when he's got it good!" Or perhaps, "If all this couldn't satisfy him, nothing can!" Exactly what I thought myself. And Bev and I were honestly troubled about my discontent even in the face of so much good fortune.

But bear with me a while longer, if you will. I think you'll be surprised to know that there is something that satisfies, something so marvelous that even one as obsessive-compulsive, perfectionistic and "thirsty" as I am can be totally fulfilled.

Before I describe that *something* for you, let me share with you what transpired following the above disillusionment with the practice.

Refusing to believe that this emptiness in my life could ever find fulfillment, I continued the search for *something*. This time I headed down the road marked "Easy Street."

I had heard the reports that one of the last reported statements of Howard Hughes was, "I'm not satisfied." I knew first hand what it was to be dissatisfied. But I could not for the life of me fathom how anyone with so much wealth could also be so miserable. So, disregarding all the dead end and detour signs, I began setting my sights on the accumulation of money, things, property and all that the world says should make one happy.

I am exceedingly thankful that I did not reach the end of my life only to learn what Howard Hughes learned. I found out in only a few years what he learned only too late. As the bank account began to grow and we began to fill our lives with "things", that old familiar companion returned to dog my heels like a shadow. The burning void was bigger than ever!

It is said that Alexander the Great, who conquered the existing world of his day, after he had overcome the last remaining power outside his domain, sat down and wept bitterly. His own emptiness cried out within him, "Is that all there is?"

I had, I reasoned with myself, dreamed some great dreams. And with a lot of hard work and perseverance many of them had come true. But all the degrees, all the professional and business success, all the money, and all the things of the world could not satisfy the consuming fire within. At that juncture I actually reached the point of saying to my own emptiness, "No more . . . That's it . . . You'll just have to content yourself with your own discontent." Through a frustrated cynicism I resolved with myself to live with my own emptiness and to be satisfied with only fleeting moments of real peace. You see, by this time even the dreams and the schemes and all the enthusiasm that went with them had long since dried up.

My life was like the mountain climber who had scaled the highest peak on earth, and there was nothing left to climb. Only the trip down.

With a cynical, "sour grapes" stoical indifference I therefore resolved to be the best therapist I could, keep the practice alive and well, and to be passively content with it all—with life. That's not very exciting, but life had lost all excitement for me.

Although this has the ring of a tragic ending, it turned out to be the beginning of the greatest discovery of a lifetime!

Looking back now it is clear that the dreams had to stop coming. The compulsive striving after attainment and success had to burn itself out. In short, everything that I could produce in my own efforts had to be proven futile and only temporary at best. And even the cold stoicism served its purpose. The ego had to begin a long, slow and painful dying process so that the "something" that had stirred my inner being for so long could reveal itself. But Self had to get out of the way to see the Truth.

What followed began one of the strangest periods of my life. Never had I been interested in spiritually oriented subjects, unless you can call humanistic existentialism spiritual. And yet I found myself drawn increasingly into spiritual things. I began reading with some interest books on Zen, Buddhism, Hindu and Eastern philosophies, and on various forms of meditation and altered states of consciousness. I even found myself integrating these ideas into our work with patients with some success.

In retrospect I can see that there was a kind of mellowing process taking place in my life that was preparing me for what was about to transform my entire life.

A growing spiritual curiosity began to dominate my thinking. I suppose that the mind becomes more attuned to higher things when the decision to get off the achievement treadmill is made in earnest. Anyway, as I began to explore this new world of the unseen something fascinating began to take place in the seen world around me. For some unknown reason I noted that my relationships with people were becoming more rewarding. I was beginning to enjoy my family to a greater degree. And I even began to notice a love for my parents that had hitherto been lacking in me. And all the while the practice continued to grow and we prospered as before.

Something unseen and very powerful was at work in my life. Something that I could neither understand nor control. And for us obsessive-compulsive, perfectionistic types, that's unnerving! What was going on?

It was as though a kind of "ripening" was taking place in me. The emptiness was still there alright, but as ripples go out in all directions in a pool, my life began to take on a new nature. Who or What was causing this incredible thing? Where was this strange phenomenon coming from that caused me to sense a love for people that I had never known before? And the question that puzzled my mind most was, "Why me?"

Logic, reason and common sense provided no answers to these questions. I explored and exhausted every avenue I could conceive of in a psychodynamic and psychological search for the key to this puzzle; all to no avail. Something was influencing my deepest and inner-most being—and I could not get a handle on "it" as hard as I tried.

As the ripening and mellowing process moved on and life grew increasingly more rich, I began to wonder whether perhaps whatever this "force" might be was the very thing that my emptiness had been hungering for all my life. Could it be, I asked myself, that there *is* something or someone outside myself—a spiritual entity of some sort—who knows the hidden need of my soul?

I *knew* that there was no God. I was proud and verbal about my position as an intellectual atheist. A personal God was, I believed, for the very young, for the very old, or for the very naive. And of course, much of my university training had supported these views and comforted me in good company.

But as I began to look around for someone, some human being, to attribute all my good fortune to, I could find no one—especially and including myself. I knew I didn't deserve such a rich life. I felt unworthy and almost guilty for having so much. And it was at that very point of unworthiness that the idea hit me like a mighty rushing wind. "Could it be . . . is it possible that there is Someone up there?" "Has all this happened in my life so that He could somehow get my attention?" "Could it be that there really is a personal God up there?"

Almost simultaneously with these thoughts I found myself looking up at the ceiling and actually speaking out loud these questions into the air. Then followed even stranger words. I said, "If there is in fact Someone up there; if You do exist and have been responsible for all the good things in my life; if you are real, then show me some sign. If you are real and do exist, then I will do whatever it is that You wish me to do."

As these words flowed easily out of my mouth there was a overwhelming sense that I had made contact with "something" or someone. It seemed almost as if I had plugged into a power outlet and the energy and power began to flow.

But at the same time my rational mind began to weigh and measure what I had said. The computer in my mind began to print out, "This is ridiculous nonsense . . . what are you doing talking to the ceiling, you fool!" And as usual, I listened to that computer and dismissed the entire experience as ridiculous and nonsensical.

That evening as my wife and I sat in our living room talking I sensed that something was not right. A tremendous force or power of some kind was approaching me, surrounding me. My wife's words seemed to fade away and "The Force" just came on like a powerful wave from off the sea. With every ounce of strength and will that I had I gripped the arms of the chair and attempted to resist. I knew that it was bigger than me and I did not want to give myself to its full control. Whatever it was, it was unknown and to be feared, I thought.

But all efforts to hold it off were fruitless. As this incredible power took hold of me what I experienced I can only call psychologically impossible, not explainable in natural (or scientific) terms.

The first impression was one of being consumed by a power that I could only identify as one of profound and infinite *love*. It was not like any human love, but was perfect and complete and directed at me personally. At the same time I can only describe what occurred next as a feeling of *returning home*. I felt as though I was in the presence of a *Father*, a perfect, loving Father and that I belonged there, in His love more than I belonged in this world where I had spent 32 years of my life. There was a sense of total belongingness as if I was created to be with Him, in love.

Mixed with these reactions were other feelings. I felt a sense of grief and loss at the same time. I felt as though I was losing an old friend—me. That I was witnessing the death of a life-long companion. The person that I had been for 32 years was slowly dying before my very eyes! But with the sense of loss came a knowledge that he had to go to make way for the new man that was being newly re-created.

There followed a sensation of a kind of decreasing and almost a "melting" of ego or self. As I found myself becoming infinitely small, I found the power of this force absorbing me, as the ocean swallows up a raindrop. It was truly magnificant!

The entire experience lasted perhaps twenty seconds, that was all. And the next thing I recall is finding myself holding my wife in my arms there in the chair, with tears flowing down my face. All I could say over and over again was, "Thank You, thank You, thank You." I was thanking a Person. A very real and very wonderful Person whom I had denied and cursed and scorned most of my life. I was thanking Someone who had just changed my personality around in seconds. Someone who had taken away every single doubt.

And I was overflowing with thanksgiving to Someone who had just entirely filled to overflowing that emptiness, that void that I have been describing to you. *It was gone!* The One who had put that emptiness in me had just filled it with *Himself!*

You see, the void was God-shaped. God, a loving Father, who wouldn't let anything besides Himself satisfy me, had revealed Himself to one of his children, to me. And the only words adequate to express my feelings were, "Thank You!"

As you can imagine, my wife, who is herself trained in psychology, witnessed all this in utter shock. She found herself married to a new person. A total personality transformation had taken place—the husband that she knew for five years was gone; he had died moments before.

As I told her about what I have just shared with you I told her that I had to have a Bible right away. A Bible—something that I had forbidden in my home—there was a driving compulsion to read it.

I opened the Bible and read a few passages and closed it. "Honey" I told her, "As incredible as it may seem all the doubts and all the questions are gone — completely!"

At the outset of this chapter I told you that my responsibility to you would not be fulfilled unless I shared something more with you. What you have just read is that something more. I offer it to you because we are both dedicated to helping humanity overcome the sorrow of mental suffering. We are colleagues, you and I, in a common pursuit. I have opened my own life to you because I believe that what has taken place in my life can in some way help you, in your personal and professional life.

Yes, this is an unlikely place to find the testimony of a "religious fanatic." That's true. But I had to put accepted protocol aside. Let me tell you why.

On September 25, 1978 at 9:00 a.m. a Boeing 727 commuter flight was approaching San Diego's Lindbergh Field. One hundred and thirty five business and professional people had boarded the flight in Sacramento and Los Angeles that morning and planned a day of work or rest in San Diego.

At 9:01 while all passengers were preparing to land and to go their separate ways, a small, single-engine plane struck the right wing of the 66-ton 727.

"Tower, we're going down." These were the last words of the 727 pilot as the 135 "souls on board" plunged toward the earth at over 280 m.p.h.

One hundred and fifty human lives ended in seconds. 135 passengers in the huge aircraft. Two passengers in the small plane. And thirteen unsuspecting souls in their homes in a quiet San Diego suburb. And not one single person among the 150 who died that morning planned to die! Not one!

Every single one of those individuals thought that they would step out into the sunshine of San Diego, California and that they would choose how their day unfolded.

But things didn't work out as they planned. Instead they stepped out into eternity!

If it is true that there is a God; and if it is true that He has planned this universe in some sort of orderly fashion, then perhaps He has designed a human life with some sort of order also. Those 150 souls who stepped out into eternity and faced their Creator face to face do not have the opportunity that we have. In this moment we have the precious opportunity to *know* where we will spend eternity should a mammouth aircraft come plummeting through our ceiling, or our heart stop beating.

Let me ask you a profoundly important question. If at this moment you should find yourself on the other side of death, do you *know* with absolute certainty how you will spend the eons of eternity? Have you given it any thought?

I believed at one time that death just brought a kind of long sleep or just a sudden thud that ended all conscious experience. But I was deluded and so terribly wrong.

Our training in human behavior and the workings of the human mind tend to lull us into a kind of sophisticated complacency. We get so caught up with explaining and diagnosing and treating that we fail to plan for something we cannot control. And eternity is a very long time!

My fellow colleague, you can *know* for certain about your personal relation to God and *know* that you have found peace with Him. You can *know* where you are going following this brief time here on earth. And you can *know* the full, meaningful and abundant life here and now through allowing Him to guide and direct your life.

Let me share four things that you need to know, the four things that He has taught me, so that the "God-shaped void" in your own life may be more than filled. It's been nearly three years now and the old emptiness and restlessness have never once returned to haunt me!

Let me share these four Truths with you and then we'll be done.

(1) "For all have sinned and fall short of the glory of God" Romans 3:23.* Every one of us has fallen short of the perfection of God. And that sin in each of us separates us from God, forever.

(2) "For the wages of sin is death" Romans 6:23. That inherent sin in us earns us eternal separation from His presence. A Holy God cannot exist with sinful man. Something has to be done about our sin condition. And no amount of good deeds or right living or psychological sophistication can help us in this regard. "The wages of sin is death."

(3) Something has been done about it, about our sin nature. Listen very carefully to these words, if you will.

"For the wages of sin is death, BUT the gift of God is eternal life in Jesus Christ our Lord" Romans 6:23.

"God made Him (Jesus Christ) who had no sin, to be sin FOR US, so that in Him we might become the righteousness of God" 2 Corinthians 5:21.

"But God demonstrates His own love for us in this: While we were still sinners Christ died FOR US" Romans 5:8. God became flesh and dwelt among us. He became our stand-in, our substitute. He is the bridge that reconciles man back to his Creator. Christ absorbed all our sin in His perfect substitutionary sacrifice on the Cross.

Is Jesus Christ the *only* way to eternal life with God? Although it sounds extreme, Christ is the only Way.

"Jesus answered, 'I am THE WAY and the truth and the life.

No man comes to the Father except through Me" John 14:6. Why the *only* way? I suppose because God chose no other way to cancel out sin except through His Son, Jesus Christ.

So our fundamental problem is sin, separation from God. The penalty for sin is death—eternal separation from God with full consciousness of that existence! And God, because of His great love for us, gave His only Son that we might live. That brings us to the last step.

(4) If Christ is the answer to all our searching, to all our striving and aimlessness, what must we do with that knowledge? You've probably heard much lately about the "Born Again" experience. The

---

* *The Holy Bible, New International Version,* Zondervan.

experience that I described for you in my own life was such an event. Of course, not everyone has exactly the same kind of feelings or dramatic conversion. But the experience is always real and life-changing. But how can it happen to *you*?

Listen to the written voice of God, from His Word.

"That if you confess with your mouth, 'Jesus is Lord,' and *believe* in your heart that God raised Him from the dead, you will be saved" Romans 10:9

"To all who *received* Him, to those who believed in his Name, He gave the right to become children of God—born of God" John 1:12,13.

Asking God to forgive our sins; accepting His Way to total cleansing from sin; making Jesus Christ Lord and Master of our life; and then receiving all the fullness and abundance that only He can give any life—that is what it means to be Born Again.

At 9:01 on that September morning 150 souls lost whatever opportunity that remained to receive what Christ had done for them. I pray that they knew Him and are with Him now.

We don't know how many tomorrows we will receive. We may not be fortunate enough to reach a good old age and then give Him what's left of our lives as some do. But we do have today!

I do not believe that it is any random event or accident that finds you reading this at this moment. God uses strange instruments sometimes to reach out to those He loves. And *He loves you!*

I leave you with the prayer that God will abundantly and richly bless your new or growing practice in every way. I also ask that this Handbook be instrumental in that endeavor. And most of all, that God draw *you* to Himself and make Himself real to *you*—and that He help you receive Jesus Christ as your Lord and your Saviour.

To those whom this material offends, please forgive me for my outspoken approach. You see, I remember what it was like being so near, so terribly near to finding out the Truth too late. *I care* and therefore I cannot be silent, not even in a book on making a private practice successful!

To you who are searching, to you who can identify with my own long journey, and to you who know personally about that aching Void, to you I dedicate this entire work. If I can be of further help to you, please do write to me. Share with me what God is doing in your own life. What an adventure is awaiting you!

And to those of you who already know Him and have experienced His serenity and joy much longer than I, to you and with you I rejoice in the certainty that He is coming again soon! *Maranatha!*

NOTE:
Comments, inquiries, personal reports of methods, plans and ideas should be directed to:

Dr. Charles H. Browning, President
Duncliff's International
3662 Katella Avenue
Los Alamitos, California 90720

THREE YEARS LATER. . . .

It's been that long. Three years working with fellow professionals to help them build lucrative practices and find new freedom in their lives. How rewarding it has been working with them through the mail in consultation, over the phone, here in the office, and especially through *Private Practice Handbook*. And to our great surprise, our non-mental health colleagues have found the *Handbook* helpful in developing their own practices; especially Chiropractors and Optometrists—the latter group showing the most interest!

We've seen many wonderful results from those who have told us how they implemented the ideas and methods in the First Edition. Many of those you read about in the last chapter. But above the satisfaction that we feel in watching others prosper and their practices fulfilling their dreams, there has been one outcome that is difficult to describe in words. That's the reactions of so many who wrote and shared *themselves* and their *lives* after seeing themselves in the present chapter.

No, we did not get all flowers! Of the many hundreds of copies distributed, we received a total of six stinging rebukes. Here's a sample:

> "I ordered a book about how to run my private practice, *not* about how to run my spiritual life!"

I had anticipated those "bricks" when preparing the First Edition. But even when you anticipate them, *brother!* —do they hurt when they land on you!!! Nevertheless, I can well understand because had I myself ordered this same book six years ago, before Someone got hold of my life and read this same "religious c———", I would have written a poison pen letter that would have wiped out half a dozen mail men (mail persons!) trying to deliver the thing. In my own case, Shakespeare was absolutely right: "Me thinketh he protesteth too much." I do hope that this is also the case with those crack shot brick throwers! Perhaps by the Third Edition we'll know?!

Anyway, I received another "brick," but they were unhappy with my writing style. . . .

> "You've got some good ideas, but your writing style is simple and juvenile. . ."

I suppose he's right, you know, uh, like, uh, well—you know. Believe it or not, throughout undergraduate, master's, and doctoral work in the university I got the reverse side of this brick, chiding me for being "to verbose" and "Browning, we know you have something to say, but we just can't figure it out for all the words on the paper!" They were being kind, and they were right, of course.

Then one day I ran across that book I mentioned in the last chapter, Flesch's marvelous classic, *"The Art of Plain Talk."* And to my surprise, he had quoted what I thought was my own dissertation (it wasn't, but it could have been). . . .

> "We are dealing here perhaps rather with a misapprehension as to the actual facts than with a confusion as to the use of terms, but the facts themselves are important in this connection because

they bear upon our views as to the line of solution....(ad nauseum...)."

Flesch convinced me that I was guilty of a "tyranny of words." But Victor Schwab, an advertising man, convinced me that if I wanted to get a message across to others, I had to KISS—Keep It Simple Stupid. He said,

"Whenever people are particularly muddled in their thinking they invent big words to cover up their confusion."

Now you know why this manual reads like a newspaper rather than the *Journal of Applied Psychology*. It's just too bad for the members of my doctoral committee, bless their patient hearts, that I found this secret out so late!

Well, enough of those bricks, let's mention the flowers!

Just the other day while opening the mail I smelled the sweet aroma of some of those flowers! Here's the letter from a therapist in Oakland, California—

"Thank you for a very helpful book on starting a private practice. I saw myself so clearly in Chapter....."

And she goes on to ask for particular help with regard to some insurance matters in her practice.

A very successful optometrist in Topeka, Kansas wrote in his second letter after reading of my own search—

"At present, I feel very frustrated because I no longer believe that inner peace, goodwill toward men, and eternal life are unobtainable. I am frustrated by my inability to achieve these. I have been praying and reading the New Testament."

One year later another letter from this same optometrist read—

"I now have more confidence and encouragement than I have ever received before....but I'm still in a dilemma as to what Jesus's message really was, uncertain whether or not he was divinely inspired and lives today, and disillusioned with prayer, I have put the matter on the mental shelf labeled 'awaiting further light.'"

Those that await usually receive!

Another Master's level psychologist said this—

"Back in 1971 God really started dealing with my life. I made a commitment to Him at that time, but I guess I was just afraid of what He might do with my life. Since then I went through a humanistic existential counseling program, started my own practice and started making all kinds of money, and I guess I am not willing to find out what God might want to do with my life now.

But when I read your book, I knew God was trying to tell me something. But I don't know if I really want to find out what."

We've received many other letters just like this one. But there is one very interesting difference in the above letter. He ends the letter with this statement—

"I don't even know why I am writing to you, you will probably never answer anyway. But my wife and I lost our little baby last year. Since then our marriage has been falling apart. It seems we just can't talk any more without ending up screaming at each other in hate. I guess I thought maybe God was trying to help us through your words. I am confused. . ."

This therapist had no way of knowing that he was writing to another kindred spirit. You see, just a few months before he wrote his letter to me, my wife and I lost our two-week old son, Adam Charles.

God's ways are indeed strange. Bringing us together at just this particular time. I could understand and feel his pain. His broken heart, and that of his wife, we were experiencing too. And our faith was also shaken and bruised for a time.

We were even angry at God for some months after Adam died. "Why would God let our baby die?" we would torment ourselves with that question every day. Why, when we were trying to please Him in every aspect of our life, why would he take him, while a baby in the isolette right next to Adam got well and went home with his Mom and Dad? Is this what it means to be a Christian? Would a God of love do a thing like that? If this is what happens to His friends. . . .!

We kept trying not to ask those natural questions, but somehow they just kept coming into our heads.

But since Adam's departure a year and a half ago, God has soothed and bound up those wounds and has begun a healing process in us. He has brought us to understand in a way we never could have before Adam, that God is sovereign and all wise, and never makes any mistakes. His ways are not my ways. His thoughts are not my thoughts. His plans are not my plans. He's God, I'm not.

Someone has wisely said that God is too loving and too wise to let one of His children shed one needless tear. This means that this tremendous hurt, this "soul-surgery" in our life was necessary, purposeful and right.

It was only through staying close to God in His Word that we were able to come back closer to Him, and stay close to each other and our other children. Through His counsel in the Scriptures He held us together while He restored our bleeding souls. And He has made us content—although we still grieve for Adam—with *His plan* and *His purpose* in this thing. And He's helped my wife and I love Him because of *who He is,* not because of what we can get out of Him or for what He can do for us. I think we once treated Him like some Cosmic Butler, Who would come running at our every call. We could only learn such a lesson from our Adam!

Three years ago I told our readers and anyone who would listen about the "only-skin-deep" God that I knew then. . . .we talked about God scratching the itch and filling the void. And all of that is still so very true and real today.

Now, however, I realize that I was only sharing part of the story, the shadow and not the substance. What I didn't know, and what I couldn't see then was this:

"For by Him all things were created; things in Heaven and on earth, visible and invisible. . .All things were created by Him *and for Him. . .*"

Colosians 1:16 ff

"Worthy is the Lamb that was slain" (for us!)

Revelation 5:12

I suppose we, in our finite minds, continue to grow in our understanding of Him who is infinite. So three years from now I'll be ready to see a new facet of His great love for us.

May He help you and me hear what He wants us to hear.

"Let him that has ears to hear, Let him hear."

A sign on a board outside a church said, "If you're tired of sin, come on in!"

Some enterprising soul, with what appeared to be a stick of lipstick, wrote underneath, "If not, call (212) 631-2487!"

I do hope you're not reaching for a lipstick. . . .and that you're tired, as I was—and that *you*, "come on in.!"

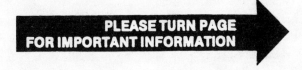

"HOW TO BUILD A PRACTICE CLIENTELE
USING KEY REFERRAL SOURCES:
A SOURCEBOOK"

Finally, you may be interested in Duncliff's new practice marketing and promotion workbook—the *"Sourcebook."* It lets the therapist pinpoint the most reliable sources of new patient referrals to the practice in his or her own area. It also gives a detailed marketing networking strategy by which to effectively approach these resources.

Many therapists become enthusiastic about promoting their own practice and make a few good contacts that result in new business to the practice. But they tend to stop there.

Other well-intentioned clinicians spend far too much time working on building a referral relationship with people who simply don't refer.

The new *"Sourcebook"* helps the therapist (1) make the business of practice promotion/marketing a regular, planned part of the operation of the practice, thus increasing practice income dramatically; and (2) helps avoid needless hit-or-miss prospecting for the best sources of new patient referrals by providing in-depth market research data pinpointing "who refers, who doesn't."

And finally, in addition to targeting the best individuals, groups and organizations to get to know, the *"Sourcebook"* gives the therapist a broad working marketing plan showing methods to win favorable attitudes toward the practice itself.

Who Refers More Patients, More Often?

The fastest way to establish a steady inflow of new patient referrals is to identify and focus all one's efforts toward developing positive working relationships with those individuals or groups who tend to refer the most people to a mental health practice. When the therapist limits his or her efforts to these key resources, the practice becomes well known by those who most need its services—and referrals naturally follow.

The "*Sourcebook*" helps the therapist zero in on these key referral sources and plan a careful sequence of contacts to build the practice clientele. Some of the Key Referral Contacts identified in worksheet forms include—

* **Community Referral Sources** . . . 81 contacts
* **Key Professional Referral Sources** . . . 40 contacts
* **68 Key Mass Media Contacts**
* **15 Important Political Contacts**
* **Over 50 Good Referral Sources in Your Present Caseload**

7 Ways to Effectively Reach Them

Once the person, group or organization has been chosen for contact by the therapist, a plan or strategy is needed by which to contact them. One method will not work with every resource person or group. The strategy must be tailored to the needs, function and personality of the target resources chosen. The "*Sourcebook*" describes a copyrighted "Referral Networking System" showing the therapist 7 ways to get the maximum attention for his or her work from the right people. Take a look at a brief outline of the "*Referral Networking System*"—

Strategy 1: Client Networking—ways to develop good referral sources from your present caseload.

Strategy 2: Shotgun Networking—making normal, everyday contacts produce new referrals

Strategy 3: Who's Who Networking—focusing on the most influential people in your community to build practice reputation

Strategy 4: Publicity Leverage Networking—using other people's publicity to increase new referrals

Strategy 5: Direct Publicity Networking—how to use the media to establish practice image

Strategy 6: Direct Mail Networking—making your announcements, letters, and newsletters more effective to stimulate new sources of practice income

Strategy 7: Advertising Networking—how tastefully done, ethical advertising can benefit any practice, large or small

Tools for Managing the Referral Process

To help the therapist gather, organize and use important facts about every new referral source developed, a new Referral Contact Tickler File system has been developed. One file card is provided for every new contact made—organizing vital information about each person or group to make the next contact more smooth and effective.

A second card file focuses on "Client Resource Data," letting the therapist pinpoint potential new referral sources from every new and existing patient or client. This can be easily incorporated into the intake procedure of the practice.

The Key Referral Tickler File system is designed as a 3 x 5 card file for easy reference, and is an invaluable practical aid to effective practice marketing.

Turning Ideas Into Referrals

The new "Sourcebook" is the therapist's hands-on master planning blueprint to convert into action the ideas in its companion volume, "Private Practice Handbook." Ideas alone do not produce new referrals. Using the "Sourcebook" each idea or strategy can be tailored to the best referral source available, and deadlines set for implementation.

Basically, this workbook gives practice promotion work order, direction, purpose and, most importantly, translates good intentions into concrete action. And that's what produces a full schedule of patients in any practice!

If you'd like a personal copy to use with the *"Handbook,"* you'll find ordering information below.

—————————————— *Clip or Photocopy & Mail* ——————————————

Reserve Order Form   *Mail To:*   **DUNCLIFF'S INTERNATIONAL**
3662 Katella Avenue, Dept. S
Los Alamitos, CA 90720

I would like to order the new companion workbook, *"How To Build A Practice Clientele Using Key Referral Sources: A Sourcebook"* to help plan and organize practice promotion activities to increase new referrals to my practice.

Please rush _____ copies to me at the address below. I am enclosing with this order a check for $9.95 plus $1.50 for postage & handling. As before, I understand that my complete satisfaction is guaranteed or money back.

Tax Deductible as a "Professional Business Expense"

Your order will be shipped within 48 hours after order received.

Please Print or Simply
 Attach Your Business Card:

NAME _____

ADDRESS _____

CITY _____ STATE _____ ZIP _____

"I have read quite a few books on establishing and maintaining a private practice. Yours by far is the most practical, informative, and inspirational ..."

—*David E. Mullen*, M.Div., M.A.
Ph.D. Candidate
Private Practice
Sarasota, Florida

"Using the ideas in this manual my practice increased by 30% in six months. I was completely satisfied and am reaching the point where my part-time practice will become full-time."

—*Kenneth B. Koffer*, Ph.D.
Fellow, York University
Private Practice
Toronto, Ont., Canada

To order gift copies of **Private Practice Handbook** *for a friend new to the business of his or her own practice, or to give as a special business gift, see ordering information on the following page . . .*

<u>20% discount</u> on all gift orders . . .

The publisher would like to help you get a friend or colleague off to a fast start in his or her new practice. Or perhaps the *Handbook* would make a good business promotional gift to other therapists in your area. If you order additional copies using this special courtesy order form, Duncliff's will give a 20% discount on each copy ordered.

If you don't want to cut out the order form, simply photocopy and mail to publisher, using the address below.

If you would like us to send the book with a personal gift card from you, please enclose it with your order and we'll include it with the book and send it direct to them. Otherwise, we'll send to you at address you list below.

— — — — — — — — — —*Simply Clip or Copy & Mail* — — — — — — — — — —

Courtesy Order Form

Mail To: **DUNCLIFF'S INTERNATIONAL**
3662 Katella Avenue, Dept. GH
Los Alamitos, CA 90720

Please send me_____ copies of *Private Practice Handbook* to be used as gifts or practice promotional items. I understand that using this order form I receive a 20% courtesy discount on each manual I order.

I am enclosing my check for _____ to cover purchase of_____ Handbooks @ $15.96 for each softbound edition; or $19.96 for the hardbound deluxe edition. I am also in-cluding *$2 per book* for postage and handling.

☐ *Please include the special gift card I am enclosing when shipping the book.*

Please Print or Simply Attach Your Business Card:

NAME_____

ADDRESS_____

CITY_____ STATE_____ ZIP_____

—*Please see next page . . . .*

If you need help . . . .

. . . . and would like personal consultation to evaluate practice promotion plans, and to receive recommendations from an experienced practice management consultant, simply write for information to:

DUNCLIFF'S INTERNATIONAL
3662 Katella Ave., P-Lab
Los Alamitos, CA 90720

NOTES

NOTES